Christian
Healing

Also by Mark A. Pearson

Why Can't I Be Me? Understanding How Personality Type Affects Emotional Healing, Relationships, Spiritual Growth. Chosen Books, 1992.

Chapter 4, "Gifts of Healing," in *The Gifts of the Spirit.* Creation House Books, 1993.

The Basics of the Faith. Latimer Press, 1994.

Christian Healing

*A Practical and
Comprehensive
Guide*

Mark A. Pearson

Second Edition

Chosen Books
A Division of Baker Book House
Grand Rapids, Michigan 49516

Published by Chosen Books
a division of Baker Book House Company
P.O. Box 6287, Grand Rapids, MI 49516-6287

Third printing, January 2000

Printed in the United States of America

Library of Congress Cataloging-in-Publication Data

Pearson, Mark A.
Christian healing: a practical and comprehensive guide / Mark A.
Pearson.—2nd ed.
p. cm.
Includes bibliographical references.
ISBN 0-8007-9221-1
1. Spiritual healing. 2. Health—Religious aspects—Christianity. I. Title.
BT732.5.P415 1995
234'.13—dc20   94-16615

For current information about all releases from Baker Book House, visit our web site:

http://www.bakerbooks.com/

This book is dedicated to my parents

The Rev. Hedley A. Pearson
and
Beverly L. Pearson

Acknowledgments

I would like to thank all those who have helped me in the writing of this book. In particular, special thanks to my colleague-in-healing Mary Shelton, who made many valuable suggestions for the whole book, but especially for the chapter on the healing of memories; and to my wife, Mary, who, in the midst of a demanding medical internship, always found time to comment on each chapter and, more importantly, give me lots of love and moral support.

Much of the material in this book was fleshed out, theologically and practically, during the seven years I was part of the fellowship of St. Paul's Church, Malden, Massachusetts. Special thanks go to two men who were then the full-time clergy of St. Paul's—the Revs. Jürgen W. Liias and Roger W. Wootton—who always provided wise, godly reflection as concepts were being pondered and ideas were being tested.

I wrote portions of this book while I was "in residence" in three different churches. Thanks to the clergy and people of St. Paul's Church, Malden, Massachusetts; the Church of St. Michael and St. George, Clayton, Missouri; and St. John's Church, Sharon, Pennsylvania, for their spiritual blessings and practical assistance.

In this revised, expanded edition, I have added at the end of most chapters several suggested discussion questions and an "experiment." The purpose of these is to make the book more usable as a healing team training manual. The questions and experiments at the ends of chapters 1–12 were thoughtfully crafted by Harry Camp, a Christian attorney from Tennessee. Harry has served his Lord faithfully for many years and has been a leading figure in the United Methodist Renewal Services Fellowship/Manna Ministries, a ministry working for spiritual renewal in the United Methodist Church.

Mark A. Pearson

Contents

Foreword

I will be honest with you. When I picked up this book to read, I intended to skim it. This rapid approach was not because I did not think Father Pearson's book would not be excellent. I know Mark as well-educated (an Oxford graduate) and brilliant, and realized that anything he writes will be worthwhile. It was just that I was swamped with work and manuscripts and thought I had best scan it rapidly and gather the gist of all he said.

Instead, I found that I was drawn into the book, and took the time to read it because, although I have had 25 wonderful years in the healing ministry myself, I found that God has gifted Mark with some important insights that I had not seen before.

In chapter 12, for example, on setting up a prayer team, he says that the person he chooses for the team does not necessarily have a healing gift! Instead, he looks for such qualities as having a strong spiritual life, being loving and being teachable. At first that surprised me. Then I realized Mark is probably right.

Another important insight I had never seen before:

The mighty works of God are not described as miracles in the New Testament, but as signs and wonders. To call them miracles would imply both that they are somehow violations of the natural order and that they are rare. Rather than violating the order of things, God's intervention in people's lives when they pray *is* the natural order.

Father Pearson does an excellent job bringing together the basic truths about healing prayer from three streams of Christianity: the sacramental, the evangelical and the charismatic/Pentecostal. What characterizes his presentation is *balance*. He is specially helpful, for instance, in presenting a brief, succinct account of the New Age movement and precisely where its dangers lie.

Whatever religious background you come from, I believe you will find *Christian Healing* an excellent introduction to the healing ministry if you are just getting started, or an important addition to your library even if you have been praying for the sick for many years.

Francis S. MacNutt, Director
Christian Healing Ministries
Jacksonville, Florida

Introduction

The twentieth century has seen a marvelous renewal of the healing ministry of the Church. This resurgence in our time of a significant part of Jesus Christ's own ministry finds a major impetus with the extraordinary explosion of Pentecostalism throughout the world, a movement maintaining that healing is integral to the evangelical message.

In the mainline churches, spiritual healing has been courageously pioneered by such persons as Agnes Sanford and Glenn Clark and respectfully promoted by the Order of St. Luke. Healing services have become a normative part of the life of many traditional churches and are included in their liturgical forms (e.g., the Episcopal *Book of Common Prayer*). Since Vatican II, the Roman Catholic Church has transformed the sacrament of unction from a rite for the dying (extreme unction) to a sacrament of healing. The charismatic renewal throughout all the churches has brought a renewed sense of the immediate experience of the Holy Spirit into the life of the believer with a rediscovery of many of the more "miraculous" gifts of the Spirit, including healing. Evangelical Christianity, though historically ambivalent about spiritual healing, has seen a wondrous opening to the biblical command to heal, thanks to the work of pastors like John Wimber. Finally, even secular medicine has become a strong advocate of the extraordinary power of faith and hope in the healing process.

As the Church rediscovers this vital part of her commission and seeks to empower clergy and laity to exercise this ministry, there are many areas of concern, both theological and pastoral. My former parish, St. Paul's Episcopal Church, Malden, Massachusetts, and the Institute for Christian Renewal developed over the years a unique training program of teaching and practicing the art of Christian healing from which this excellent book has evolved. It is both a theological-biblical primer on the principles of Christian healing and a practical instruction manual on the art of spiritual healing, useful to individuals and especially parishes.

I pray it will be a most useful resource for Christians to discover and share the awesome joy of healing in the name of Jesus.

The Rev. Jürgen Liias
Church of the Advent
Boston, Massachusetts

1

The God
Who Heals

One of the great blessings to occur in the life of the Church in recent years is the revival of the ministry of healing through prayer. While as recently as thirty years ago relatively few churches conducted healing services, now many do, and the number is growing. Truly this ministry is being restored to its rightful place in the life of the Church.

And why not? Healing is at the very heart of who God is. The Bible tells us repeatedly that God is all-powerful and all-loving. These words remain platitudes, and God remains an abstraction, until they are applied to real situations. To say that God is love and yet not see Him at work in people's lives is a cruel contradiction. The God we worship is not an absentee landlord but a loving, caring Father who ministers to His children at their points of need. Sometimes the need is for healing.

The second Person of God came to earth in human form, in part, to make more widely known and more easily available the various blessings of God. Not surprisingly, therefore, healing was a major part of the ministry of Jesus. His very name means "salvation," a word connoting more than forgiveness of sin unto eternal life. The word literally means "wholeness." Our Lord's earthly ministry was to minister this wholeness in every area of our lives. God invested Christ in us when He sent Him to die for our sins. And He intends to keep up His investment! Put another way, God, who loved His enemies so much as to send Christ to die for us (Romans 5:8–10), will certainly not abandon us in our needs now that we are His friends.

The ministry of healing through prayer leads people to God. Some, like the nine lepers who did not return to give thanks (Luke 17:17), will always "take the healing and run." Others, having received the healing, fall in love with the Healer. For many this is the first time God has seemed real.

To be sure, there were healings in Old Testament times, but they were occasional and done through a few extraordinary prophets. But then, because of Jesus' message and ministry, healing became widespread and happened through the prayers of simple fishermen and other ordinary folk. In Old Testament times an incident or two of God's healing would be reported, then none for a long time. But from Jesus' day onward, healing was deemed a regular part of the life of the Church.

The Gospel writers describe our Lord as going about teaching, preaching *and healing* (Matthew 4:23; 9:35; etc.). One-fifth, or 727, of the 3779 verses in the four Gospels have to do with healing in some way or other, a significant amount considering all the various doctrinal and ethical matters that had to be addressed.

Jesus trained His followers in the ministry of healing and sent them forth to heal in His name (Matthew 10:1, 8). In the Upper Room Jesus told them they would continue this ministry after His return to heaven, when He said, "Truly, truly, I say to you, he who believes in me will also do the works that I do. . . ." (John 14:12).

In the Acts of the Apostles we see the young Church effectively ministering healing just as Jesus had done (see, for example, Acts 3:1–10; 8:7; 9:33–34; 14:8–10). Their ministry of healing helped authenticate their message. Although their Holy Spirit-inspired and -empowered preaching won many to the faith, many others were convinced only when they saw the signs and wonders that attended their ministry (Acts 8:4–7; 9:32–35). While other religious leaders might merely have talked about what they believed, the followers of Jesus demonstrated graphically that in Christ a new order had begun. What they said—that the Kingdom of God had been inaugurated through Jesus of Nazareth—was happening for all to see.

The mighty works of God are not described as miracles in the New Testament, but as signs and wonders. To call them miracles would imply both that they are somehow violations of the natural order and that they are rare. Rather than violating the order of things, God's intervention in people's lives when they pray *is* the natural order. We may not understand this natural order, but just as many of the inventions we now take for granted were once thought out of the realm of the natural order, so, too, we may someday understand how God responds to our prayers.

Similarly, those who have walked with the Lord for even a short time begin to see that the number of "coincidences" increases dramatically when God's people turn to Him in believing prayer. William Temple, Archbishop of Canterbury during the Second World War, used to say that the more he prayed, the more the "coincidences" happened. Healings—and other blessings—are not rare, except to those who do not ask God to go to work in human lives.

Thus, we describe the manifestation of God's healing power as signs and wonders. A sign does two things: It gives both information and direction. We look for signs when we travel to tell us how far a distant city is and which of the various roads we should take to get there.

Healing, as with other signs of the Kingdom, gives us information as to what God is like and points us to where abundant life is found. The healings, important as they are, point past themselves to the Healer Himself, whom to know is eternal life and to serve is perfect freedom.

Healings are wonders as well. As we see a loved one helped by divine intervention, or a life set free from a bondage or an illness, no matter how many times we have seen God at work before, we marvel at both His majestic power and the fact that God, "who has so much to do," would take the time to care about ordinary persons in need.

The healing ministry of Christ and His Church is not, therefore, an optional extra. It is one of the ways people get from God the help they need so very much. God wants His people made whole, and people today, in spite of tremendous advances in medicine and psychology, still need the direct intervention of God for healing.[1]

How wrong is the statement we sometimes hear that the Church's ministry of healing might be O.K. "if you're into that sort of thing." To keep the ministry of healing from God's people because it happens not to interest the leaders of a given congregation is as much spiritual malpractice as it would be medical malpractice for a hospital to refuse to treat heart attacks because its staff preferred only to treat pneumonia.

This is not the attitude Jesus wants us to have. As a beloved Christmas carol puts it, Christ is "ris'n with healing in His wings." He left us a great trust. But why the need for healing in the first place? If God loves us so much that He will send healings, in other words, then why did He ever allow us to get sick?

The answer is that the human race has been given free will and that our misuse of this—corporate and individual—has brought on ourselves, others and the whole created order the various consequences of sin. These include sickness in body, soul and spirit. In fact, the human race has been under a curse since Adam's sin.

We can see the extent of the curse in the early chapters of Genesis, where we read how Adam and Eve disobeyed God: In the aftermath of their sin, they hid themselves from Him—a sign of their spiritual sickness and sense of estrangement from God (Genesis 3:8–9). Adam blamed his wife for the temptation—illustrating emotional sickness and disintegration of relationship (Genesis 3:12). Adam and Eve became subject to physical sickness, pain and death—which we likewise suffer (Genesis 3:16, 19). Cain killed Abel—illustrative of societal sickness (Genesis 4:8). The ground yielded thistles and thorns—demonstrating how even creation became skewed through human sin (Genesis 3:17–18).

The healing Christ offers is as extensive as the damage done, or, to quote another carol, as "far as the curse is found."

There is spiritual healing through forgiveness of sin and the promise of eternal life, offered to all and experienced by those who receive Christ as Savior (John 1:12). Our chief sickness is alienation from God. In Christ, the curtain of estrangement is torn down between us and God (see Mark 15:38) so that we may become His sons and daughters, live in fellowship with Him now and enjoy eternal life in heaven with Him when we die.

There is healing for the turmoil within people and between people as the Lord sets the captives free emotionally and behaviorally. As evangelist Tom Skinner once put it, Christ wants not only people taken out of the slums, but the slums taken out of people.

There is physical healing through science and through the ministry of the Church, sometimes instantaneous, sometimes gradual.

There is societal healing as God works in the corporate hearts of groups of people and of nations.

There is a renewing of the earth as God restores what we need to survive. Total environmental and cosmic healing will come when, in the new heaven and earth, the lion will lie down with the lamb and disorders and disasters of the environment will be put in order. Until then, creation stands on tiptoe waiting for it (Romans 8:19-22).

To be sure, these are all foretastes for now. At some point in the future when Jesus Christ returns to make the heavens and earth new, the very presence of sin, with all its harmful consequences, will be removed. At that point believers in Christ will experience healing perfectly. As for now, while we do not experience healing perfectly, *we can experience healing substantially.* To accomplish this in us, God works in several ways.

Four Ways God Works Healing

One, through skill and science. God has given us minds to use to unlock the secrets of creation. When God told Adam to subdue the earth (Genesis 1:28), He was not telling him it was permissible to pollute or despoil. Rather, He was saying that one of the ways we discover His provisions for us is through human skill and science. Although these are imperfect—doctors, nutritionists, trainers and counselors make mistakes and lack complete knowledge—they are intended by God to bless us and promote our well-being.

Luke is honored as "the beloved physician" (Colossians 4:14). Nothing in Scripture indicates that Jesus wanted Luke to abandon his craft and simply pray for his patients. Paul instructed Timothy to "use a little wine for the sake of your stomach and your frequent ailments" (1 Timothy 5:23). Although using a little prayer for healing would also have been appropriate, Paul encouraged Timothy to make use of a substance that, when taken in moderate amounts, can have a healing effect.

Two, through the rites, clergy and sacraments of the Church. Services of worship often are occasions for physical, emotional and spiritual healing, even if they are not intentionally healing services. We will discuss this more extensively in chapter 9. I will just say for now that the sacraments, like

Jesus, incarnate (or flesh out) the spiritual reality of God in material ways. The bread and wine of holy Communion do not just symbolize the benefits of Christ's broken body and shed blood; they bring these realities to us. The oil of anointing (James 5:14) is not just a visual aid. It is a "delivery system" for God's healing. To be sure, we can go too far and turn sacraments into superstitions. But we must not neglect the sacraments as a means that God uses to bring us His healing to us.

Three, through the various spiritual gifts God has given the Church. Any number of people have been specially gifted by God to heal in a way that is dependent entirely on His grace and not on human skill or science (1 Corinthians 12:9). Others have received gifts that augment or assist the ministry of healing. Often, as with so many things of the Lord, the people specially gifted to heal are not the ones we would expect. (We will look at this in chapter 10.)

Four, through the prayers of all Christians. The Church ministers healing corporately through the members' love for one another. In addition, any individual Christian, whether or not an elder of a church or the possessor of healing gifts, can be used to pray for the sick. Jesus said, "These signs will accompany those who believe . . . they will lay their hands on the sick, and they will recover" (Mark 16:17–18). (We will examine how God can use individuals in a ministry of healing in chapters 12 and 13.)

These last three ways in which God works to minister healing could be given the descriptions *Catholic, Pentecostal* and *evangelical.* It is easy to see why. Catholic Christianity stresses the importance of liturgical rites, orders of ministry and the sacraments. Pentecostal Christianity gives special emphasis to the various spiritual gifts, which are often manifested in powerful and spontaneous ways. Evangelical Christianity, in addition to holding before us the primacy and authority of Scripture, upholds the ministry of all believers.

Three Streams, One River

Half a century ago, a bishop in the (interdenominational) Church of South India named Lesslie Newbigin described in his book *The Household of God* (SCM Press, 1947) how important it is for the Church to incorporate *all* the riches God has given it. He saw three streams—Catholic, Pentecostal and evangelical. In order to let the Church be the mighty river God wants it to be, the three streams, so often kept apart, must flow together. As a bishop in the Church of South India, which was the product of the merger of many denominations of different traditions, Newbigin saw the possibility of the streams coming together and feeding each other.

Sadly, though offered this mighty river, most Christians have contented themselves with just a rivulet. We in the healing ministry would do well to resist this tendency. We need all of the four ways mentioned above for healing, for two reasons:

One, we dare not insist that God go about His work only in the ways we prefer while refraining from helping us in ways we do not. If we truly believe God is the sovereign Lord of our lives, we will receive what He wants us to have *in the way or ways He wants us to have it.*

Two, each one of the four ways, when held together, keeps the others from going off into imbalance.

The mind orientation of skill/science and of preaching the Word needs the balance of the mystical other-worldliness of sacrament and of spiritual gifts. The mind is a wonderful gift of God, but it is only one way to know Him, hear Him speak or receive His blessings. God is also known, heard and enjoyed through our innermost being, sometimes called the spirit. God comes to us in ways beyond our understanding, as anyone who has encountered Him in worship or in a sunset can attest. Were this not so, people of modest intellect, or the retarded, or anyone whose mind is tired, would find fellowship with God hampered.

Encountering God in such mystical ways, however, has its dangers. We must make sure that any so-called experience of God conforms with what He has revealed in Scripture. Otherwise we will be at the mercy of accepting anything as long as it "feels good" or seems "other-worldly."

Additionally, the stress on one's personal faith in God, so emphasized in evangelical Christianity, has to be balanced by a similar stress on the sovereignty of God. While our grasp of God is important, so is His grasp of us. When our faith is weak, it is good to know that through the sacraments and spiritual gifts, God is reaching out to us, even apart from our ability to respond. Our faith ebbs and flows. How good it is to know that God remains constant! While personal feelings of faith are subjective, the sacraments and spiritual gifts are objective, available to us even when we are weak.

Yet without a personal relationship with Christ, we can easily become passive recipients of ministry. We might receive a specific blessing at a point of need, while not knowing or knowing well Him who is the source of all blessings. If our personal relationship with God in Christ is nonexistent, we are still dead in sin.

Furthermore, the kind of individualism seen in each-member ministry or in persons exercising the spiritual gifts has to be balanced by the sense of the corporate as represented by skill/science and by a catholic sense of the corporate Church. Professional practitioners of medicine or nutrition are not free to act in accordance with their own whims, but must act in accordance with generally accepted standards of medical science or nutrition. Their understanding and adherence to such principles is monitored and they are accountable to their fellows. The Church over the centuries has formulated theology and liturgy according to what people of many cultures and temperaments heard God saying. They worked to preserve the truth and hold their teachers accountable. This tended to weed out individual quirks of understanding.

Yet neither science nor the Church is infallible. Science is often improved when a solitary voice challenges that which has been accepted. Reformers, often speaking alone, have repeatedly called the Church to rediscover parts of the biblical message that have been misunderstood or neglected. When a local congregation is indifferent or even hostile to the ministry of healing, sometimes one lonely voice "crying in the wilderness" opens the way for the good news of healing to be heard and experienced.

The "routine" of science and sacrament has to be balanced, moreover, by the fresh, new and often dramatic inbreaking of God as individual Christians minister through the spiritual gifts. The love of God is ever fresh. He who does not make two snowflakes alike ministers to His people in a variety of creative ways. God who made the exciting phenomena of earth and sky often ministers in ways that are stupendous.

Yet God is also a God of order. We do not have to wonder if summer will be followed by autumn, or if gravity is operative on a given day. God, too, wishes us to know that His healing is regularly available through skill/science and through sacrament. Dramatic actions, when God is their author, can be thrilling, but sometimes people seek not the Lord but the phenomenon. And one can be so busy focusing on the uniqueness of how the ministry is taking place that the content of the ministry is lost.

All the streams, therefore, are needed, because they help keep each other and us in balance.

Even though each stream is given by God and of great importance, individuals sometimes turn off to one or another of the streams. This can happen for several reasons.

Reasons for Not Accepting "Full Gospel" Christianity

One, bad theology. If the only way a particular stream of Christianity has been presented to you is in the context of bad theology, you may indict that stream itself and not the bad presentation of it. A physician may describe the way our bodies function or the possible cause and cure of a particular illness. That is science. The physician may go on to talk about the existence of God or what constitutes moral decency, and may try to convince us that this, too, is science. It is not. It is theological and philosophical speculation masquerading as science. If we do not catch this subtle shift, we may turn off to science in general and deprive ourselves of a source of help.

If the way we have encountered the sacraments is in the context of a theology that makes it sound as though the sacraments are magical ways to manipulate God, we might reject the sacraments entirely or relegate them to mere symbols.

If the people who have spoken to us about spiritual gifts also try to convince us that for us to experience them, we must have a dramatic encounter with the Holy Spirit and immediately start speaking in tongues, we may not agree with their theology and reject the whole idea of spiritual gifts.

If those who tell us about the ministry of each member of the Church also assert that there is no special role for the scientist, the clergy or those with spiritual gifts, we may reject the idea of lay ministry on the basis of this other assertion.

Two, wrong practice. Sometimes the theological understanding of the stream is correct, but the way in which it is carried out is wrong. Science can be presented in an arrogant manner. The sacraments can be offered in a way that is dull and boring, or in a way that looks like hocus pocus. The spiritual gifts can be used in a way that burns people up, not warms them. Lay ministry can be incompetent.

Three, foreign "packaging." It is a fact that we often judge something more by its cover than by its contents. Each of us has a certain way we like our Christianity to be packaged culturally. This depends on our upbringing, our personalities, what we value in music or art, and so on. If the style in which one of the streams is offered is not valued, we may reject the stream itself.

If the only way we can picture psychiatrists, for example, is as beady-eyed, intense little men with goatees and Viennese accents, all therapists may be dismissed by negative association. Or if our image of a sacramental church is an ethnic, blue-collar Roman Catholic parish, what we think about that subculture will strongly influence what we think about the sacraments in general. Or if when someone mentions spiritual gifts and what comes to mind is a rural Pentecostal tent meeting, then we may reject the spiritual gifts if this is not our style. Or if the term *lay ministry* implies pouring out our private business to our peers who will then spread it around town, then we will not let anyone except "the professionals" help.

Four, prejudice. Our prejudice against "experts," Roman Catholics, Pentecostals or the idea of our waitress or auto mechanic ministering to us may keep us from receiving the help from God we need.

If we can overcome these pitfalls, we will be the richer for it. Additional sources of grace will be available, for our sake and for the sake of those to whom we minister. And if discovering other streams via the ministry of healing has proven a blessing to us, we can integrate these streams into all other aspects of our walk with Christ and come to enjoy a fuller, richer discipleship. Over the years I have seen many move to a full Gospel faith because the ministry of healing was presented to them in a full Gospel way.

While skill and science, the sacraments, the spiritual gifts and the ministry of fellow Christians may be the means God uses to bestow healing, it is vitally important to remember the source of all healing is Jesus Christ. We must ever keep this before us for at least two reasons.

Jesus, the Source of All Healing

First, seeking (and receiving) a healing without seeking and finding the Healer is settling for much less than is offered and needed. The most important healing anyone can ever have is to be healed spiritually by reconciliation to God through Jesus Christ. Kathryn Kuhlman once said, "I don't care if I never see another physical healing as long as people keep coming to Jesus Christ. That's the greatest healing." Assembly of God pastor Tommy Barnett points out, "Miracles are so mighty that often we are tempted to glorify them rather than get on with the work of the Kingdom. Miracles are meant not to dazzle us, but to help us carry out the great Commission of Jesus Christ."

This is not to say, of course, that physical or emotional healing is not important. Kathryn Kuhlman continued her own gifted ministry of healing. It is, however, to place things in proper priority. As a historic Communion liturgy puts it, "Through faith in His blood, we . . . have remission of our sins and [then, and secondarily] all other benefits of His passion." Or to quote a Scripture made popular by a contemporary praise song, "Seek ye first the kingdom of God, and his righteousness; and all these things shall be added unto you" (Matthew 6:33, KJV).

For this reason, a ministry of healing is better entitled a ministry of *wholeness*. We want for ourselves and others not just to look at the specific physical, emotional or spiritual problems, but at whole lives in light of what God wants for us. Whether healing comes through medicine, a "miracle" at a healing service or help through pastoral counseling, we are doing a disservice if we do not bring our entire lives before God—and help others do the same.

Second, seeing Jesus as the source of all healing is critical, given the rise of the New Age movement. Many methods of healing are now being offered that are either based on humanistic techniques or else that seek help from spiritual powers or beings. At best these are foolish, for they press people to look for cures and not for wholeness, and to seek it from sources that cannot give wholeness. At worst these methods put people in touch with entities that are not surrendered to God, that are condemned by God and that seek to harm the creation of God, however friendly they look at first. Although people sometimes receive healings through these spiritual beings, often the end is worse than the beginning since these beings are spiritually, emotionally and physically harmful, and now have special access to those who invited them to come and heal.

There is much we do not know about the ministry of healing. We will have many questions for God when we see Him face to face. But for now, our less than perfect knowledge should not stop us from making use of this rich ministry of blessing called healing through prayer. God wishes to bless us more than perhaps we had once expected. As He blesses us, let us love Him for who He is, and ask Him to use us as His blessing to others.

Discussion Questions

1. List New Testament examples of restoration to wholeness.
2. What does all this reveal about God? About yourself?
3. Of what significance is healing to the Church?
4. List the different types of ailments.
5. List four basic procedures for healing.
6. Discuss the limitations inherent in each procedure.

Experiment

Select a person with whom to share that you are studying a book on Christian healing. Tell the person you need help—that you would like to pray for someone to be healed, and ask if he or she will cooperate. If so, ask the person to tell you of a physical problem or broken relationship that needs healing. Pray and invite the person to pray also. In a notebook begun for this purpose, record information similar to that kept by a doctor, including at least the date; the person's

name; the ailment; how you prayed; what you told God; what
you asked God; what, if anything, you felt God saying to you;
your physical posture and that of your "patient" during prayer
(if you laid your hands on this person, and if so, how); if the
patient prayed also; if you agreed to have additional sessions;
and any discernible results.

You may want to make an appointment for further prayer.
Keep a meticulous record. After about four weeks talk with
the person; evaluate and record the results. Critique your
procedure. This will help you measure your growth as you
continue in the study of this book.

2

Why Did Healing Decline?

The ministry of healing occupied an important part in the theology and experience of the Church in the first three hundred years of her existence. In the fourth century, however, a serious decline took place and the focus shifted. Healing was not taught nearly as much, nor was it often experienced. Something had changed. It was not that God had intended for healing to be part of the Church only in her infancy and then to disappear once the Church had gained a firm footing. Rather, other factors came into play that caused the decline in this ministry.

These factors, having nothing to do with the purpose of God, are still with us. It has often been said that history repeats itself. As we examine the various reasons for the decline in the ministry of healing in the fourth century, we see striking parallels as to why the ministry of healing is downplayed or even rejected by many in the Church today.

Why did healing decline in the fourth and fifth centuries and why is it not a major part of the life of the Church today? Let's look at the reasons.

The Church as Part of the Establishment

Prior to the fourth century, Christians were persecuted for their faith and many were martyred. The only ones who identified themselves with Christ and His Church were the ones who meant business. Those early disciples believed the Christian message and knew that nothing else could compare even remotely with it. To them it mattered not a bit what others thought about them. Mockery and persecution did not deflect them from their belief that what Christ taught was true, what He promised would happen and what He commanded should be done. Thus, they received the promises about healing and obeyed His instructions to minister it to one another.

In the fourth century, however, much of the Church lost this fervor. In 313 A.D. the Emperor Constantine's Edict of Milan gave official tolerance to Christianity. Although a brief return to persecution occurred later in that century, before long Christianity was not only tolerated but became the established religion of the Empire. The Church was soon flooded with nominal believers for whom the radical centrality of Christ was secondary to social acceptance and career advancement.

The result? For many, the promises of success in careers took precedence over the promises of Christ in healing (and other things); the call to make it in the world was heard over the call to do the hard work of the Lord; and the desire for being deemed respectable more than outweighed the embarrassment of being deemed zealous.

Are things so different today? Are there not a variety of lesser motivations for church membership than the Gospel call to die to self and live to Christ? I know of many churches in which a committed core of believers desires to receive the blessings of Christ and follow Him wherever He leads but is thwarted by those who do not want their church to challenge them to have a relationship with God, to make demands on their lifestyles or to do those things that would make them look odd to their peers.

Many want just enough religion to make them look respectable or feel good, but not enough to force them to change. The ministry of healing startles nominal Christians in much the same way as Jesus' walking on the water startled the disciples in the boat. A rabbi who goes around telling people to be good threatens no one. But when that rabbi walks on water, those watching know immediately that if they are seeing what they think they are seeing, the old ways are gone forever. They are faced with three logical choices: deny what they see, passing it off as a hallucination; try to kill that rabbi in a desperate attempt to cling to the status quo; or respond in faith, significantly advancing their commitment. One thing they cannot logically do is shrug the event off.

Methodist leader John Wesley noted the correlation between the decline of the various gifts of the Spirit and the deadness of the Church.

> The causes of their decline was not as has been [commonly] supposed because there was no more need for them. . . . [T]he real cause was: the love of many, almost all Christians so called, was waxed cold. . . . [T]he Christians were turned heathen again and had only a dead form left.

False Zeal and Fanaticism

While we strive for a true, self-surrendered zeal for Christ, some fall into a false, out-of-balance zeal. Even prior to the fourth century was the unfortunate appearance of the Montanists, a group in the Church that emphasized the miraculous workings of the Holy Spirit far out of proportion to everything else in the faith. Later, as nominal believers started to determine the tone of worship, some of those who were keen for the Lord reacted further still. We recall the misplaced dedication of one Simon Stylites. Simon, recalling the Scripture "At the name of Jesus every knee should bow" (Philippians 2:10), climbed a stylite, or column, and recited the Lord's name over and over again, genuflecting as he did so. For many, including many of the truly devout, such excesses tended to have an overly tempering effect. The powerful move of God and the dramatic operations of the Holy Spirit became somewhat suspect, even when done in scriptural balance. Many dedicated believers became cautious, and the ministry of healing (as other good things) suffered.

The unfortunate excesses of a small minority in the charismatic renewal of today have made some people similarly wary. In addition, certain emotionally troubled individuals who have gravitated to the ministry of healing have discredited legitimate expressions of Christian healing in the eyes of some. I often find myself spending more time telling people what I do *not* mean by Christian healing than what I *do* mean. Obviously the bizarre and the unusual garner the headlines and make those of us who want a balanced healing ministry suspect. There are just enough examples around of churches divided and individuals harmed to make many who believe in Christian healing overly cautious. While I would hope to convince such people that the answer to one extreme is not flight to the opposite extreme, some will conclude that the benefits of Christian healing are not worth the risk.

Asceticism or Rigorism

While some reacted to the growing nominalism of the fourth-century Church with a false zeal, many others adopted a rigorist posture. Some fled to the desert, there better to confront the devil and purify their souls. Rejecting many of the creature comforts of the city, they felt free to focus on becoming like their Lord who had nowhere to lay His head. In contrast to this, healing, especially physical healing, seemed a self-pampering compromise.

Today many are reacting to expressions of Christianity that seem to be self-indulgent. The wealth of the Church in this country—in the face of world poverty, racism and oppression—strikes many as obscene. People have commented, "We have too much as it is; why should we ask God for yet more?" Others have stated that what we need is revolution, not pietism.

The enticements of the "prosperity gospel," encouraging people to grab onto as much comfort as God will provide, strike many as bearing little resemblance to the model of Jesus, the "Man for others." In short, prayers for healing seem, to some, selfish.

I maintain that receiving a blessing often equips and motivates one better to be a blessing to others. Had it not been for my sudden healing from chronic bronchial asthma in 1979, I would not have been able to make several ministry trips to those third world places where a severe asthmatic response would have been likely. Part of the motivation behind my going on these trips, moreover, was gratitude to God for His healing me.

Additionally, asking God for a much-needed healing is different from asking for material wealth. And for some, the inability to ask God for help is not a sign of embracing evangelical poverty but of either proud self-sufficiency or neurotic self-abnegation.

A Philosophy that Deems the Body to Be Less Important than the Soul

In the fourth century, a popularly held philosophy was Neoplatonism. This view, which gained a strong influence on the life and thought of the Church, held that the body was irrelevant to the all-important soul. What God really cared about was our inner spiritual life. It was, after all, the soul that lived on. Why bother with the body, which would perish anyway? This belief failed to take into account the numerous examples of our Lord's healing bodies, or the fact that Christianity is based not on a Greek body-soul dichotomy but on a Hebrew psychosomatic unity. It failed to understand that Christianity affirms the resurrection of the body, not just the immortality of the soul. It forgot that God deemed the physical creation "good" (Genesis 1:31) and that the problem with the world is sinful rebellion, not physical existence.

Some people today understand these things intellectually, but maintain an often subconscious separation between the physical and the spiritual. "Don't pray for my arm to be healed; pray that I grow to be more like Jesus," I was once told. No matter how hard I tried to convince this person that one could indeed pray for both, the lingering notion prevailed that any blessings the body received would somehow be at the expense of the soul.

Sickness as a Punishment for Our Sins

As the western part of the Roman Empire crumbled in the fifth century, the Church took on a pessimistic, otherworldly stance. As life became rougher and the so-called Dark Ages began, people were encouraged to look for blessings chiefly in the world to come. Sometimes pagan tribes, with their views of a vengeful, wrathful God, were only partially converted as they were incorporated into the Church. Their views influenced the attitude that no one should ask God for anything except His tolerance of us wretched children of Eve. For a long time physicians were not allowed to treat the sick until the priest had first heard the sick person's confession, for it was felt that sickness was a direct punishment for sin. Whatever recovery might ensue was secondary to getting back into the good graces of God.

While few would formally hold such notions today, many still have a vague feeling that we are too unworthy to ask God to heal us. We may avail ourselves of medical science, but we should come to God only to beg His mercy, not seek His blessings. One man questioned me thus: "God heal me? But I don't deserve a healing, given all I've done wrong." It did no good to remind him that Jesus came for the sick, since the well have no need of a physician (Mark 2:17), or that the whole point of the Gospel message is that God wishes to bestow grace on the undeserving.

The Split of the Church

In the first few centuries of the Church, much interplay of thought existed between her Eastern (or Greek) and Western (or Roman) halves. Nevertheless, Christianity in the Western part of the Empire tended to be more matter-of-fact and oriented toward duty. As long as the Church had a sense of oneness and East and West kept constant communication, the two differing emphases were kept from becoming too extreme. Eventually, however, as East and West increasingly went their own ways, two different styles of Christianity emerged. In the Roman West, Christianity meant obedience to God's laws, not mystic communion. Save for a few mystics, it lost the Eastern understanding of personal encounter with the numinous. Healing, more akin to the Greek half of the Church, was less at home in the Roman half.

In today's Church we see similar splits into groups that have little influence on each other. Pietists and social activists, traditionalists and renewalists, intellectuals and mystics—all reflect various aspects of the whole. But the various streams come together all too infrequently to form that mighty river of comprehensive, full-Gospel experience of which Bishop Newbigin wrote. Individuals growing up in one Christian subculture may live their whole lives without firsthand knowledge of other expressions of the faith. Certain aspects of Christian life may actually be considered to belong to one or another of the Christian subgroups, having nothing to do with us and our part of the Body of Christ.

Forty years ago in the Episcopal Church, someone interested in anointing with oil for healing was immediately deemed an "Anglo-Catholic." Today that person is immediately labeled a charismatic. Given the fact that anointing with oil for healing is a sacrament of the Church with its own service in the *Book of Common Prayer,* an Episcopalian believing in this ministry should simply be called an Episcopalian. More importantly, with the weight given this ministry in Scripture, such a person should simply be called a Christian. Such a ministry, in other words, is "generic" Christian.

Most of the Christian churches of today's West—whether fundamentalist or liberal—are still centered in correct performance of duty, however that may be defined. It is still difficult for many to conceive of the faith as personal encounter with God through which lives are transformed and healed. And there is little regular communication between those churches and the others—largely charismatic or Pentecostal—in which healing is a regular part of church life.

The Cult of the Saints

"Healing miracles," when they did happen, were associated for many centuries with great figures like St. Francis of Assisi. Given their unique sanctity, it was not hard to understand healing occurring at their hands. It was considered presumptuous, however, for anyone else to attempt to perform such works, or to expect them to occur in general. Thus, in spite of our Lord's direction that all of us should do the works He did (John 14:12), the experience of healing was restricted to those fortunate enough to be helped by a "saint."

Such an attitude remains with us today. Many Roman Catholics who save up for a trip to the shrine at Lourdes, France, hoping to be healed, deem foolish the suggestion that a healing could occur in their own parishes. Others petition a deceased holy person for help (witness the prayers to St. Jude regularly printed in newspapers), but will not ask a fellow Christian to minister healing to them. Many Protestants flock to healing crusades conducted by well-known evangelists, not realizing that God can also use the prayers of the folks in their own church.

Yes, of course, there are those specifically gifted in healing (1 Corinthians 12:9), just as there are those specially gifted in preaching, teaching, counseling and so on. But while we thank God for and make use of their ministries, we are not to deny ourselves what God can do through all members of the Church, nor are we to deem it presumptuous to think He can also use us. Every congregation should have a regular ministry of healing. All Christians should pray with expectation for the sick to be healed.

A Bad Use of Scripture

Since the early days of the Church, there have been those who get from Scripture a message far different from its plain, simple meaning. Whether this stems from blinders put on by the intellectual outlook of the day, or from a proud desire to be clever, or from a refusal to believe something they themselves have not experienced, or from a desire to rewrite Scripture to their own liking, the result is the same—a portion of God's Word lost to His people.

In the early centuries of the Church, passages were sometimes "spiritualized"—that is to say, a word was thought to be a symbol or even a code for something else. When it came to healing, some saw Gospel references as parables, not literal accounts. They taught, for example, that the man healed of blindness was not *physically* but *spiritually* blind. I wonder how much of this was an excuse to cover the fact that the Church at that time lacked the faith to believe and experience healings of physical blindness?

Another blow to the ministry of healing came when Jerome translated the Bible from Greek to Latin (the Vulgate edition), which was, in his day, the common language of the educated of the Western Empire. The Greek *sozo* (save) and *soteria* (salvation) are rich words speaking of deliverance from a wide spectrum of danger or harm. In the narrow sense, the words mean deliverance from the danger of eternal damnation, much as people today use the word when they say, "So-and-so went to an evangelistic crusade and got saved." That is not, however, its only meaning in Scripture. The word can mean "healed," as the context of James 5:15 indicates. Here, however, Jerome rendered the word as "save" (in the narrow sense of the term), not "heal." Thus, a key text for the Church's ministry of healing was lost to the Western Church. Coincidentally, the sacrament of unction—anointing the sick for healing—was being transformed slowly into the sacrament of extreme unction—the "last rites" preparation for death.

In today's Church, the proverbial "man in the pew" is bewildered by the various theologies—which go in and out of fashion rapidly—that serve to undermine confidence in God's written Word. It seems that every time we turn around we are told that Paul did not write a particular epistle attributed to him, that Jesus did not utter this or that word the Gospels quote Him as saying, that our Lord's doing of one or another deed was the invention of the early Church, that a given verse does not mean what it says or that it no longer applies.

While many of God's faithful continue to shout, "Thanks be to God," when a lector concludes a reading of Scripture with "The Word of the Lord," and while they continue in many different churches to see what is promised in Scripture play itself out in their lives, many others are confused. And in their confusion they miss out on much of what God wants for them. It is difficult to prepare for battle when the trumpet sounds an uncertain note (1 Corinthians 14:8). It is difficult to have confidence in wielding the sword of the Spirit, which is the Word of God (Ephesians 6:17), when one is told the equipment is faulty.

Besides theologies that undermine confidence in Scripture as the trustworthy Word of God, there are theologies that, while claiming to uphold the authority of Scripture, misinterpret it. Job is often cited as a person who grew in sanctification because of what he suffered in his sickness. Yet Job 1:8 tells us he was "blameless and upright," without peer on earth. Scripture also tells us (e.g., Romans 8:17) that we must suffer with Christ. This is often interpreted to mean that we should endure our pain or disease stoically. Yet the sufferings Jesus endured (e.g., Matthew 16:21) were persecutions, not illnesses.

Yes, healing declined in the early centuries of the Church and continues to be in decline in some segments of the Church today. But that is due to the ignorance, fear, laziness and sin of its members, not the desire or purpose of God. When church members submit to God's will and trust His promises, healings happen. May God give us His grace to be part of the restoration process of this much-needed ministry.

Discussion Questions

1. Identify modern examples of the spirit of
    a. The Church as part of the establishment
    b. False zeal and fanaticism
    c. Asceticism or rigorism
    d. Neoplatonism
    e. Sickness as punishment for sins
    f. Brokenness in the Body of Christ
    g. The cult of the saints
    h. Use of Scripture to deny healing
2. What has been the greatest obstacle to your own participation in the healing ministry of the Church?

Experiment

Select a person as at the end of chapter 1. Ask him or her three questions and record these in your healing notebook:

1. Do you believe the Church should be involved in the healing ministry?
2. Why or why not?
3. Why, in your opinion, is healing in the Church so rare?

3

Objections and Answers to the Ministry of Christian Healing

Healing is a significant part of the Gospels, a regular component of the life of the early Church, a sacrament of the Church and a reality experienced by many people today. In spite of this, objections are lodged against it even by some in the Church. I am happy to say that each of these objections has a solid answer. Anyone raising objections should find the roadblocks to belief removed.

Objection #1: With all the problems in the world, isn't being concerned with healing selfish?

Look at it this way: Isn't an individual's sickness one of those problems in the world? To be concerned with personal needs does not mean one is concerned *only* for oneself. Many people are not concerned with helping others—nor are they able to be—until their own problems are dealt with. Many individuals, out of gratitude to God for healing them, give themselves in service to others in a way they would not have considered had Jesus not healed them. (Note Jesus' call to Peter to manifest his love toward his Lord by serving others—John 21:15–17).

Don't those who make this objection seek medical help when they are sick? If they do, why isn't *that* selfish?

Objection #2: Aren't there frauds and money-grubbers in the healing ministry?

Certainly, but point to a profession or calling where that is not the case! We read periodically about a physician who has bogus credentials or who, in spite of several serious blunders, is still practicing medicine. Do we reject the whole profession of medicine because of those persons?

While the televangelist scandals focused on a few individuals who lived in luxury, most ministers of healing are either unpaid volunteers or, if Christian ministry is their full-time work, are paid very little. We might, for example, compare the cars driven by doctors, lawyers and business executives with those driven by most clergy. This is not to say that these others should not be paid well in light of their educations and long working hours. It is to say that clergy also put a lot of time into education and hard work, and they are paid a lot less.

Objection #3: Healing is so rare. Why get people's hopes up only to disappoint them and hurt them emotionally and spiritually?

Who says healing is so rare? Stories abound, some with physician's statements included or told by physicians themselves, of people being healed through prayer. Often to declare that "healing is rare" says more about how little investigation the objector has done. I have heard people state flatly they knew of no one who was ever healed through prayer, when I knew several in their own communities whose healings were dramatic and lasting.

Even if healings were rare, that would be a statement about what currently is and *not about what is supposed to be*. If healing is rare, could it be traceable to a lack of vital faith on the part of the Christian community? Often revival, renewal or reformation occurs when a remnant few in the Church study the promise of Scripture and the experiences of the Church in previous periods of fidelity and start praying for whatever is missing to occur again.

As for emotional or spiritual hurt, we can encourage people without setting them up for hurt. Physicians and therapists acknowledge how important in the healing process is one's belief in the possibility of getting better. Don't physicians encourage people, with the same possibility of emotional hurt if the patient is not cured? Whether done by physicians or healing team members, an encouragement to believe in the possibility of getting well can be accomplished without manipulation or excess. Part of the purpose of this book and numerous training programs in the ministry of healing is to ensure a good and growing number of ministers of healing who are capable, effective, balanced and humble.

We also need to ask how much damage is done by the opposite extreme. How many fewer healings would take place if the physician or therapist counseled a patient regularly not to expect anything to happen? Yet how many in the Church counsel people regularly not to expect anything from prayer? Such people are sharing their own doubts and lack of experience, not the truth of Scripture and the historic experience of the Church. No wonder healing in those places is rare!

One Sunday I filled in for a priest who was away. At both services I preached on healing. After the eight o'clock service, four women out of the seventeen people who had been present related that they had been healed through various ministries of healing in the area. Each woman shared in a whisper after making sure no one else could hear, apparently believing she would be deemed odd for making such a claim! "Are you saying people in this church would think you odd for believing that one of the sacraments of the Church actually works?" I asked. "Yes," each one responded.

I wonder how many more in that congregation might have experienced healing had there not been such a climate against sharing what God wants to do for His people.

Objection #4: Wasn't healing just for the purpose of getting the early Church going, and not to be expected today?

Jesus ministered healing out of compassion for hurting individuals (Luke 17:13; Matthew 9:35–36), and to symbolize and effect the breaking in of God's kingly rule on earth. Although some who were healed became disciples (John 4:46–53, 9:38), healing was not a come-on to get the ball rolling. Jesus' compassion does not change. He is the same yesterday, today and forever (Hebrews 13:8).

The decline in healing did not occur because Jesus withdrew an inducement to faith; it occurred because the Church, having eventually become established, cooled off in fervor. The progressive unfolding of God's compassionate, kingly rule will continue until the Lord's return.

Often those who so gullibly state that healing was withdrawn once the Church got going overlook one significant fact: Healing continued! Healing died down, *but it did not die out*, and it died down for the reasons we have already examined, not because God withdrew it. As Church history illustrates, whenever vital faith flowered, healing—and indeed all kinds of divine blessings—became much more in evidence.

Further, we find no time limitations on the ministry of healing set in Scripture. When Scripture says, "These signs will accompany those who believe" (Mark 16:17), there is no phrase adding, ". . . until such-and-such a time." When

James exhorts the sick person to call for the elders of the church (5:14–15), he does not hint that this is a limited offer.

First Corinthians 13:9–12 is sometimes misunderstood to mean that when the founding of the Church or the writing of Scripture ("the perfect") was completed, the various gifts of the Spirit ("the imperfect") would come to an end. These interpretations are faulty. The Church, with all of us imperfect people, can hardly be seen as perfect or complete. And although the Scriptures are perfect and complete, we are not; we continue to need the gifts of the Spirit to help us understand and minister.

Many commentators believe that a more accurate translation of *When the perfect comes* is *When the perfect one comes*— that is, when Jesus returns. Then and only then will we see "face to face" and "understand fully." Then and only then will Jesus make the new heavens and new earth, eliminating all disease. Until such time as the Lord returns, we need all the gifts and operations of the Spirit, including the ministry of healing.

Objection #5: Doesn't healing lead to easy Christianity? Doesn't Jesus want us to bear our crosses?

In one sense, why *not* easy Christianity? Jesus came to give us abundant life (John 10:10). The Lord, our Shepherd, gives us green pastures and still waters and He restores our souls (Psalm 23:1–3). The attitude that we should feel guilty for being blessed is psychologically unhealthy and theologically unsound. God does not bless reluctantly. He blesses in abundance, as the Bible indicates (Matthew 7:11; James 1:5; 2 Corinthians 9:8).

As we are blessed, God invites us to work for the betterment of humanity, the building up of His people and the extension of His Kingdom. Being healed frees us to do our tasks. When Jesus healed Peter's mother-in-law of her fever, she got up and waited on them (Mark 1:30–31). To be sure, some will receive God's blessings but never join in the cause. Like nine of the ten lepers Jesus healed (Luke 17:11–19), they receive their healings and go their way. Should we therefore stop ministering healing because some presume upon it? Should we require people to sign up for service before we offer God's help? If we follow the example of Jesus, the answer is a resounding *no*. We hope, we pray and we encourage those blessed by God (in healing or in anything else) to become partners in ministry. Some will not, but many will. When it comes to bearing one's cross (Matthew 16:24), the context is the persecutions one suffers for standing firm for Christ, not enduring illness. If it were otherwise, then why did Jesus heal people? It would have been contradictory. Did Jesus ever tell a sick person that illness was a good thing? Although God can bring good out of anything, including illness, Jesus saw illness as an enemy to be defeated, not a friend to be embraced.

Once again we would ask the objector if he also refuses all medical attention. If the answer is no, then what happens to this objection? If we should not seek healing through prayer because God wants us bearing our crosses of sickness, why should we seek a medical removal of those crosses?

Objection #6: If we establish a healing team, doesn't that imply that some people have gifts and others don't? Doesn't it set up an elite?

Each believer, according to Scripture, is given one or more gifts for use in Gospel service (1 Corinthians 12:4). These are to be used (1 Timothy 4:14; Romans 12:6). Those whose gifts are not in the area of healing have gifts in other areas. As a church establishes a healing team, it should also establish other ministries if it does not already have them, and encourage all the members to take part. It is true that some have gifts of healing and others do not, just as it is true that some can preach, counsel, play or sing music, evangelize or teach Sunday school, while others cannot.

Any ministering group or individual could, of course, succumb to pride. Part of the ongoing supervision of the healing team by those in leadership is to encourage both confidence and humility. No, we should not wait until we are free of pride before we minister—otherwise, no one would ever minister anything. Rather, to be preferred is the attitude of Cliff Barrows toward Billy Graham when Dr. Graham's ministry was just beginning in the early 1950s: "Lord, if You keep him anointed, I'll keep him humble."

Objection #7: Isn't healing associated with spiritual fringe groups? We've seen healing done in bizarre ways.

Some groups in the Church have overemphasized one aspect of the Church's message, just as some have deemphasized other aspects. Some groups have overemphasized the dramatic and spectacular, the miraculous and otherworldly. Other groups have stressed the rational, virtually ruling out anything supernatural. The response to those groups that wrongly minister healing (or, indeed, anything) is not to turn away from it but rather to do it better and more wisely. Would we, for example, refuse to eat just because there are obese people? Would we rule out dieting because of the excesses of anorexics? The key, of course, is balance.

Dr. Charles Hummel's phrase *fire in the fireplace* (the title of an excellent book on the history and theology of charismatic renewal) has been very helpful to me over the years. According to this analogy, the fire represents the present-day experiencing of God's rich activity in the life of believers. This includes answered prayer, the gifts of the Spirit, a personal relationship with Him, enthusiasm for God and so on. The fireplace is careful biblical scholarship, the doing of things decently and in order, the consensus of the faithful over the centuries, the structures and rules of the Church and so on. The fire and the fireplace need each other! A fireplace without the fire (the danger established, traditional churches often fall into) may be beautiful, cultured and safe, but it is also cold, dark and powerless. The fire without a fireplace (a danger in Pentecostalism) can do much, but it can also burn the house down. The answer, obviously, is to build fires in the fireplaces and fireplaces around the fires. It is in this way that a healing ministry should be conducted.

Objection #8: Why should we have a separate ministry of healing? Doesn't God know who is sick already and doesn't He heal as He chooses? Aren't people sometimes healed by receiving Communion?

Yes indeed, God heals in a variety of ways, including sovereignly with no input on our part. But we have a separate, intentional ministry of healing for two reasons:

One, we are told to. In James 5:14 the sick in the Church are told specifically to send for the elders who will anoint them. Jesus sent His disciples out to heal (Luke 9:1–2). While our Lord did many things, healing is one that is distinguished from others. Since our Lord's example and direction and the Scripture's command include healing, who are we to ignore or disobey?

Two, a healing ministry makes intentional that which may occur otherwise only coincidentally, and specific that which is general. God instructs us in a lot of ways but we still have classes teaching the faith. God ministers to our problems but we do not rule out pastoral counseling. God exhorts us in many ways but we still have sermons. So, too, with healing. While there are many avenues by which God ministers healing, we need an intentional ministry of healing, a ministry in which healing is the central theme, the chief focus.

Objection #9: Didn't God use healing through prayer then because medical science had not advanced to the place it is now?

First, physicians understand that the etiology (cause) of the majority of sickness is emotional/spiritual in whole or part. In these cases, while physicians treat symptoms, medical science is useless to cure root causes. How many people do we know who have come away from their physicians shrugging their shoulders, saying, "He said it was stress"? Many physicians, referring to their patients, have said to me, "They need you more than they need me."

Nor is the solution to be found in psychological counseling alone. People face many problems because their lives are not in order as God has established it. As Blaise Pascal pointed out, we have a God-shaped void in us. We will try to fill that void with all sorts of things, some good, some not good, but nothing will fill it except God. As St. Augustine put it, "Our hearts are restless until they find their rest in Thee, O God." I do not deny the value of psychological counseling, but sometimes it, too, treats just the symptoms.

God has made us to live in personal, obedient relationship with Him. As we depart from that relationship through ignorance, laziness or willfulness, we suffer. God is not harming us for this; we are harming ourselves. Any form of healing—by medicine, counseling, nutrition or even religion—that does not center in God and His will is inadequate to make people whole. It is often inadequate even to make them physically well.

Second, although medicine has come far, especially in the last hundred years, there is much it cannot do. Antibiotics can do much but the common cold is still with us. Medicine is a good friend and part of the multifaceted approach to wholeness God provides, but it fails miserably as an infallible, all-providing master.

Objection #10: Isn't healing anti-scientific?

First, many nurses and doctors believe in and practice Christian healing in addition to their work in medicine. For them, prayer and medicine represent two interwoven strands, a much stronger cord.

Second, just because something cannot be proven in a laboratory experiment does not mean it is false. Many things that are true and dear are proven by other means. Can we weigh six ounces of patriotism? Can we produce the scientific formula for love? I was once with a group of people that included the mother of a boy who had been charged with cheating. The mother loudly protested her son's innocence. "But how do you know?" people asked her. "Because I know Tom," she said. Infallible proof? No. But the margin of error may be no greater than that in so-called scientific experiments, which are not always infallible either.

Scientific experiments rarely explain how or why certain events always seem to work in a certain way, only that they do. A laboratory scientist once told me, "We don't know why this medicine seems to produce good results in patients. But in about seventy-two percent of the cases it yields noticeable improvement. So, since there seem to be no bad side effects, we use it." I would ask that no more "proof" be required of healing. If all we can say is that many people experience noticeable improvement by praying with believing Christians—often when medicine or surgery has not helped—then fine! Why should we ask of Christian healing greater proof than we do of medicines or medical procedures?

Third, a few experiments have demonstrated the reality of prayer in the process of healing. Dr. Randolph C. Byrd, a physician on the staff of San Francisco General Hospital, decided to conduct such an experiment. He had a computer divide the names of 393 patients admitted to a coronary care unit into two sections, equal in terms of illness and likelihood of recovery. The names and problems of the people in one section were sent to intercessory prayer groups. The second section was not prayed for in this way (although doubtless some of the people were prayed for by friends and loved ones). No one in the hospital knew who was in which group, lest there be any compromise of the integrity of the experiment. After a certain time period elapsed and all the relevant data were collected, a comparison was made. This medical conclusion was drawn: Prayer to God has a positive impact on the healing and recovery of patients admitted to a CCU. (This is documented in the *Southern Medical Journal,* July 1988, pages 826–829 under the heading "Positive Therapeutic Effects of Intercessory Prayer in a Coronary Care Unit Population." An abstract of this article, as well as briefer summaries of other scientific studies, appears in Appendix 6.) Given this and other evidence, could we not validly reverse the question and say: Cannot the biases of some physicians hurt the recovery process of their patients by their unscientific prejudice against prayer for healing?

Fourth, during the last few decades there has been a profound shift in the philosophical underpinnings of science. While still believing in the validity (within its proper place) of scientific experimentation, few people now hold to a Newtonian-Cartesian view of "fixed laws of nature." The universe is seldom seen anymore as a machine operating within specific rules, most of which we know. Rather, the universe is seen more in spiritual terms, and observers are humbled by how much we do *not* know. As John Polkinghorne expressed it in *Science and Creation:*

> The very transition from the naïvely objective world, as perceived by Newton and Maxwell, to the elusive quantum world of Heisenberg and Dirac, is a tale of the often reluctant recognition by physicists of the strangeness of what actually is. If encounter with the physical world can so sharply revise our understanding of what can rationally be said about its nature, it would scarcely be surprising if the pursuit of the divine required openness to the unexpected.

Recent scientific discoveries and theoretical postulations have discredited, at least among some of the learned, belief in a closed, mechanistic universe with no room for divine intervention. The view of science held by the proverbial "man in the street," however, is often from the pre-Einstein "dark ages." In the days of Copernicus and Galileo, it was the Church that needed to be corrected by the discoveries of science. Today, ironically, when it comes to a belief in the direct intervention of God in human lives, it is science that is finally catching up with the Christian faith. (For a succinct statement of the issue, see Appendix E, "Natural-Supernatural Distinctions," in Charles E. Hummel's book *Fire in the Fireplace: Charismatic Renewal in the Nineties*. For a more thorough treatment, see *The Galileo Connection: Resolving Conflicts Between Science and the Bible* by the same author.)

Objection #11: Isn't a healing ministry likely to disrupt the good order in our church? Our service is long enough as it is without adding more!

Much depends on what is meant by *disrupt* and *long enough*. If someone is fearing wild, out-of-control zealots or services that go on and on, then I can understand the objection. I am not advocating that!

But if the objector really means that he wants a Christianity that makes no demands on him, that does not interfere with his life or is confined to one hour (and no longer!) on Sunday morning, then I would say he woefully misunderstands what Jesus' call to discipleship is all about! Jesus did not come to be fourth in our lives behind the things we really like. He came as Lord. As the experience of the rich young ruler shows, Jesus offers only one category of discipleship—*committed* discipleship (Luke 18:18–23).

Yes, a healing ministry will cause some disruptions. An effective ministry of healing will attract people who are hurting physically and emotionally. Some of them may dress strangely, act oddly or smell bad. But didn't Jesus come for these (Luke 5:30–32; 7:36–50)? And isn't part of our task as a community centered in Him to reach out and welcome into our midst such as these (James 1:27; 2:5)? A local church is a community responding to God's call—called out from the world, called to faith in Him, called together as a body and called forth to do His work. It is not a gathering of the self-righteous who want "God on retainer fee" or who want God to give sentimental feelings on demand.

Yes, as we claim more of our privileges as believers and own our duties as disciples, the service of worship will grow longer. But those who have tasted the beauty of the Lord and surrendered to Him want it that way. To someone who hates baseball, being dragged to a game can be agony. But to someone who likes it, a game that goes into extra innings is a bonus!

A Final Point

The objections examined above can be honest difficulties on the part of committed disciples. These people rightly do not wish to rush into anything while there are roadblocks in their minds. I hope we have seen that we need to take these objections seriously, and that there are answers to them.

Other objectors do not really want the roadblocks removed. As one man put it, "If God heals, then God is real, and if God is real, He probably wants me to change. I do not want to change; therefore, I wish to keep Him at arm's length. I come to church because I enjoy the music, I meet interesting people and it's good for the kids. But I do not want God to be at the center of my life. Anything that may indicate His power and reality, or anything that reminds me of any claim He might have on my life, is too threatening. Therefore, healing or any other kind of spiritual fervor is to be blocked."

I must admit, I seldom hear such an honest, articulate statement as this man gave on why some oppose healing. Yet it is the attitude, to a greater or lesser degree, consciously or unconsciously, held by many people in the Church. While respecting them as individuals, we cannot let such faithless objections deter us from starting or expanding the ministry of healing (and anything else the Lord wants us to do). The program of the Church must be based on the revealed will of the Lord and the agenda set by those who wish to know and do His will, not by those who do not.

Discussion Question

State in your own words how you would respond to a fellow church member who raised each of the eleven objections stated in this chapter. If you are in a group, you might even consider role-playing.

Experiment

Block out at least twenty minutes of private prayer time. Take at least five minutes for quiet, thoughtful, verbal thanksgiving and praise. Read Isaiah 53:1–9 slowly until a thought arrests your attention. Stop and ask God for enlightenment on that thought. (If you finish reading without stopping, start over and read more slowly and thoughtfully.) Record your thoughts, meditations and conclusions.

4

Why Are Some People Not Healed?

The obvious fact is, not everyone ministered to is healed. So the question that comes to mind is, Why not?

It is a good question. Some try to duck it, but that is foolish. If the ministry of Christian healing is nothing more than a pleasant but ineffectual ritual, we should stop it immediately. It would be dishonest to continue and harmful to the emotions and faith of those we have deceived. If, on the other hand, there is something to this ministry of healing, if God actually does wish people to be healed, we need to press on to identify and remove whatever barriers are blocking the healing from taking place. Look at a medical analogy. If a person has a medical problem and one series of tests does not yield information as to the identity and cause of the illness, does the doctor stop or does he or she run further tests? If one kind of medicine or treatment proves ineffective, do we give up trying to get well or do we try something else?

There are a number of reasons why a person ministered to is not healed. (This fact alone should keep us from making snap judgments or giving simplistic, across-the-board answers.)

1. A Wrong Diagnosis of the Problem

While God sometimes heals a foot when we pray for an arm, or honors a generalized prayer of "Lord, please bring Your healing; You know what the need is," it is often important to diagnose the problem and its root cause. We see this approach reflected in the apostle Paul's statement that sometimes he prayed in the Spirit and sometimes with the mind (1 Corinthians 14:15). When he did not know what to pray, in other words, he employed the gift of tongues, praying from the depths of his being but without any knowledge of the content of his prayers; while on other occasions he prayed with his rational faculties well-informed.

When time allows, a conversation with the person to whom we are ministering can help us ascertain the problem and its root cause(s). In addition, we should spend time asking God to give us supernatural discernment, for it may be that we cannot know what the problem truly is unless God tells us. When we do not have the luxury of lengthy conversation before ministering to a sick person, such as at a public service of healing, we can pray for discernment while the ministry is being carried out.

We should always remember the dangers of attributing every problem to only one factor and of emphasizing only one aspect of healing. Sometimes a person's problem is traceable to unrepentant sin, sometimes to a biochemical disorder, sometimes to a bad emotional experience in one's youth, sometimes to a bad diet, sometimes to demonic activity and sometimes to several root causes. Healing painful memories of the past will not set free a person who needs to repent of a certain sin, nor will deliverance from evil spirits help someone who needs to alter his diet. Although we should not push this point too far, many evangelical and fundamentalist churches tend to see every problem as sin-caused and every solution as repentance; many Pentecostal and charismatic churches tend to see every problem as demon-caused and every solution as deliverance; and many liberal churches tend to see every problem as psychological/emotional and every solution as counseling or inner healing. If we have diagnosed incorrectly, we will often be ineffective in prayer and can even do harm.

2. Limiting God to One Method

God has many and various ways to bring us to wholeness. If we try to limit Him by insisting He heal us in a particular way, we might block a healing from happening. Remember the story of Naaman the Syrian whom the prophet Elisha told to bathe in the River Jordan in order to be healed (2 Kings 5:1–14)? We could well imagine the shock to his pride for a Syrian military commander to have to wash in a Jewish river. But he did, and he was healed. Had he insisted on a method other than the one God told Elisha to use, he would have remained ill. To cite another example, Timothy's stomach troubles were alleviated by moderate drinking of wine, not by prayer (1 Timothy 5:23). I believe this is why Jesus varied His methods each time. He healed someone so he or she would center on Him, not a method.

Some Christians rule out confession of their sins; others see no value in nutritional programs; a few rule out doctors; others refuse to go to healing services. In my experience, if someone refuses to use a particular legitimate method of healing because of pride, it may well be that God will insist on that method as the—or at least a—key to healing, because pride may be the real root problem.

Remember, the ministry of healing is better and more fully described as a ministry of *wholeness*. In order for a person to be whole, God must be sovereign over that person's life. A stubborn refusal to cooperate with God in the manner in which a healing occurs may be symptomatic of the need for a spiritual healing.

3. Counteracting God's Work

If we are praying for healing but indulging in things that hurt us (bad diet, lack of exercise, letting emotional hurts eat away at us, holding onto a root of bitterness), we may be blocking the healing or else reinfecting ourselves.

Several years ago I had an ongoing stomach problem. At each "team prep" meeting before our Friday evening healing service, I asked our team to pray for me. They did and the problem went away . . . until Monday afternoon. The next Friday they would pray again and I would be healed again . . . until Monday afternoon! This went on for weeks until somebody suggested we pray for divine wisdom. After a few minutes in prayer one of the team members received a "word of knowledge" (that is to say, information about something that comes directly from God; see 1 Corinthians 12:8). "This may be nothing," she said, "but what is coming to mind as we pray is a picture of a giant coffeepot. Mark, how much coffee do you drink in the course of a day?" I was surprised—shocked, actually—when I added up the number of cups! God was not punishing me or removing my healing. I was counteracting His work.

4. Holding Onto Sin

Closely related to this is the refusal to let go of a particular sin or attitude that may block wholeness. Although it is obvious that persevering in sin blocks our fellowship with God—and therefore our wholeness—sin can also harm us physically.

I once ministered to a man who was contemptuous and abusive of store clerks. On those days that he ran an errand during his lunch hour—and inevitably got into an argument—he came down with a headache during the afternoon. While aspirin alleviated the symptoms, it also masked the cause. He consulted pharmacists for stronger medication. One of them—with whom he had an argument—tried to point out that the answer was not in a pill, but the man did not want to discuss it. Finally, when the pain got much worse, he was ready to listen. By God's grace he was able to face the problem, ask forgiveness of the many people he had wronged and take steps to change. Eventually the arguments ceased—and so did the headaches.

The psalmist noted, "There is no health in my bones because of my sin" (Psalm 38:3). And as we see in the Gospels (Mark 2:5; John 5:14), Jesus' ministry of healing often involved forgiving sins. (See chapter 5, "Sin, Sickness, Repentance, Healing.")

Increasingly, articles are being published both in medical journals and in the popular press demonstrating the relationship between sickness and the inappropriate handling of emotions. Bitterness, resentment, anxiety, inappropriately expressed anger—all of which Scripture calls sin—besides harming others, harm ourselves, spiritually, emotionally and physically. While this is not a license to tell people their faults indiscriminately, we can follow the Lord's leading and confront people lovingly but firmly with sin and its consequences, to themselves and to others.

Some people, operating out of a misunderstanding of what it means to accept and affirm others, refuse to make the connection between sin and sickness, repentance and healing. This is not because they doubt that the connection exists— the evidence of it scripturally and medically is overwhelming—but rather because of an attitude of permissiveness, or a codependent need of people's approval, or a theology that lets us do whatever we want regardless of what God has said or all three of these.

There is, to be sure, a wrong way to confront, a way that is judgmental, self-righteous and condemnatory. Jesus ruled this out when He said, "Judge not, that you be not judged" (Matthew 7:1). But there is a right way, a way that is discerning, caring and helpful. This is what Jesus meant when He told His followers to "judge with right judgment" (John 7:24). The popular term today for judging in a right way is *tough love*. It is the secret behind an "intervention" to confront a substance abuser with his addiction, and the accountability in which AA members hold each other. (See Appendix 8, "May Christians Judge?")

5. A Secret Desire to Stay Sick

There are people who would rather stay sick because their illnesses give them power over others. I once heard a mother tell her teenage daughter, "You can go out Friday night with your friends if you want. But just remember, they don't have a bedridden mother as you do, one who took care of you when you were little, one who needs you now." That woman was using her illness to manipulate her daughter, and indeed the entire family. Physicians had said repeatedly that although her symptoms were real, there was no physical cause for them. She was sick because she wanted to be sick, because it gave her power.

Other people desire to stay sick to have an excuse to avoid work, responsibility or good behavior, to attract pity or to be the center of attention. I remember how much more quickly I recovered from an illness when my mother told me, "I don't care how sick you are, you will no longer get away with that kind of behavior!" Jesus' perceptive word to the man at Bethesda was, "Do you want to be healed?" (John 5:6).

Others desire to stay sick because somewhere along the line they have come to believe that they are unworthy of health, of love, of anything good. This can be traced, variously, to parental upbringing that demeaned or abused, to neuroses of various kinds, to a theology of a punitive, vengeful God, to an overdose of the hard knocks of life, or to other causes. They just cannot believe that things could be better. Anything good that comes their way is pushed aside. Even the thought of being healed—and the new lifestyle it would bring—is scary to them. As one poor victim of this thinking once said to me, "I'm only happy when I'm unhappy." This secret desire to stay sick might be conscious or it might be buried deep down inside. But it is real and keeps some people from becoming whole.

This is not to say we do not have a ministry to such people. Of course we do! But it is to help them see either that they do not have to stay sick or that their sickness, far from warranting their being excused, warrants their being confronted. This attitude must be one of compassion and genuine understanding of the repressive faculty of the psyche and of neurosis. In doing so the sufferer must not be made to feel ashamed of needing his illness as a way to cope with the emotional traumas of life. It was what allowed him to survive emotionally until he could be brought to a different way of living that allows him to be healthy.

6. Not Seeing Healing as Gradual, Progressive

Sometimes God works gradually. We see this in Scripture with a blind man who was healed in two stages (Mark 8:22–25).

Sometimes the healing is gradual because several pieces of the puzzle need to fit together in a certain order. I ministered to a woman who had a number of serious problems, all of which were rooted in an abused childhood. I ministered inner healing until her growth into wholeness eventually plateaued. At that stage I had to shift from inner healing and start dealing with her anger toward her abusers. Forgiveness had not been possible in her until then, but from a certain point onward no further inner healing could take place until she started to forgive. Then we went back to work on inner healing.

During her childhood she had sought solace in a few foods that are nutritious enough in proper amounts but can be harmful if a diet is centered in them. She eventually became healed enough emotionally to let go of them, but then had to learn about nutrition. As she rearranged her diet, certain physical problems went away. The healing progressed, it seemed, at a pace she could handle and integrate into her life. It was a long time before she was healed of the major problems, physical, emotional, spiritual. We worked hard, but it was well worth it.

While thanking God for and marveling at the powerful, dramatic, instantaneous healings I witness at large healing services, I often wonder if the immediate removal of a painful physical problem does not sometimes short-circuit this gradual process of going deeper into a person's life and bringing before the Lord all the pieces of the puzzle. (This danger is eliminated if the person, besides attending big healing rallies, is also receiving ongoing discipleship training or spiritual direction.)

Sometimes the healing is gradual because God is using the healing process to work in the lives of other people.

I was privileged to be part of a large healing service for a few years in the mid-1970s at St. Timothy's Episcopal Church in Catonsville, Maryland. Led by the Rev. Philip C. Zampino, this service attracted several hundred people each week and many healings took place. One evening a young girl, totally blind, was brought to the altar rail by her father. Father Zampino ministered to her and there was some slight improvement. Near the end of the service at the altar call, which afforded people the opportunity to receive (or rededicate themselves to) Jesus as Lord and Savior, the girl's father came forward. His conversion seemed real (and subsequent events proved it to be both genuine and lasting).

For several weeks he brought his daughter to the services. Each week her eyes got a little bit better. And each week her father—who was taking in all he could in terms of his new relationship with the Lord—grew spiritually. Then one week he could not come. He asked his wife to bring the girl. At the altar call she went forward. Soon the three of them were in church every Tuesday night. Other family members started noticing both the growing physical improvement in the girl and the profound change that had come over her parents. They started coming, too, and some of them found the Lord. The girl continued toward full sight, and the revival in her family spread.

I often wonder what would have happened had her healing occurred in another way. This is not to say that all these conversions could not have happened had the healing come instantaneously. They may well have, but possibly not. The point is, sometimes God allows something to unfold gradually and we should trust His sovereign wisdom when it does.

7. Healing Is Not God's Immediate Will

It could be that in the short haul God is using the illness for a purpose, perhaps to get our attention or the attention of someone else. Perhaps it is to remind us of our mortality or teach us what is important in life. How many people have recovered from a brush with death to reorder priorities in their lives? How many relationships have been strengthened when an illness forced people to look at what really matters? Perhaps God has urgent things to do in us before attending to our physical or emotional distresses.

However true these things may be, we must be careful not to overdo this point. If God is allowing the illness to continue for a reason, we need to do everything possible to find out that reason! If God wants us to learn a lesson, we need to learn it, and not just remain sick. Then, once the lesson has been learned, the needed change implemented, the new attitude owned, the new behavior begun, we should expect the healing to occur. God will not usually keep us ill forever.

When a lesson is learned, a lesson is over. God has many other ways to effect our continuing education!

According to Victor Frankl, a therapist imprisoned in a Nazi concentration camp who lost his family to the Holocaust, suffering can be tolerated only when we can find meaning in it. The challenge for sufferers is to find a purpose deeper than the hurt itself. When we are sick or when we minister to someone who is sick, we need to direct effort toward learning whatever lessons await us as we pray for our healing. Otherwise, should healing not come, we may turn bitter toward God, toward life or toward others.

8. An "Illness unto Death"

If God is taking a person home through an "illness unto death" (John 11:4), our ministry should not be as much for restoration to health as it should be for the spiritual (and, secondarily, emotional) preparation for death. Has the person made peace with God by receiving Jesus Christ as Lord and Savior? This is crucial. Where we will spend eternity is the most important matter we will ever face; the opening of the Kingdom of heaven to all believers was the chief reason God the Father sent His Son to earth (John 3:16–18). However uncomfortable it may be to them and to us, we must speak clearly about eternal destiny, for the repeated teaching of Jesus is that not all will go to heaven when they die. How grateful I am that I did so with my maternal grandfather shortly before his death, and that he is now eternally safe in Jesus' arms!

Next, have they reconciled with loved ones? Are wills drawn up? Is there any other "unfinished business" that needs to be done?

Yet at the same time, we do pray for their physical wellbeing. I have seen many instances in which the patient remained ill but was relieved of pain and discomfort, and died peacefully and lucid in conscious fellowship with God and loved ones.

What about those cases when we are not certain whether it is an illness unto death or not? It may be obvious with someone who is elderly, but what about someone much younger who suffers from a so-called terminal illness? Should our efforts be toward spiritual preparation for death, or for physical healing?

The answer is both, but it takes a careful balancing of the two. We may have to contend with the denial of family members—and even physicians—who cannot face someone's death and who selfishly think it wise that the sick person "not be told" of his condition. In point of fact, many people nearing death know or suspect the seriousness of their conditions and want someone—anyone!—to talk with them about it. While we certainly want to express hope, we do not want to be swept up into the game many play, denying the severity of the illness. (We are under absolutely no obligation to go along with family or medical staff admonitions not to tell the person of his condition.) We do not want our conversations about death, on the other hand, and the necessary preparations for it to dash faith and hope for healing.

Let me illustrate how we can minister in that balanced way by telling you the story of someone I ministered to, a young woman I will call Kristi, who had terminal cancer. Kristi knew she was very sick. Fortunately, no one was hiding this from her. Her parents asked me to minister to her. As I was not certain Kristi was part of this request, I started by asking her if she would like me to talk with her. She said yes. Wanting to come in at her emotional level, I asked Kristi how she was feeling.

"Terrible, Father," she said. "It sounds like I'm going to die. I don't want to, but some days the treatments make me so sick, I'd like to die and get it over with."

We talked about her relationship with the Lord to make sure she understood the way of salvation. I discovered that she was trusting Jesus Christ as her Lord and Savior. With that most crucial issue resolved, we talked a bit about God's love, heaven as a place where there is no pain, and so on. We talked at some length about what unfinished business might be between herself and loved ones and worked out some plans as to what to do. As I noticed she was tiring, I knew I should be bringing my visit to a close.

"Kristi," I said, "we've been talking about your preparation in case you are going to die soon, but I don't know that this is what's going to happen. I don't know everything about why God does things one way one time, another way another time. But I have seen God heal people of cancer like yours. Will you pray with me for your healing?"

"I can't," she said. "I believe God can do anything, and I've seen answered prayer, but I've never seen anything like this happen."

"Well, Kristi," I replied, "if I can't pray *with* you, I'd like to pray *for* you right now. And I'm going to get a number of 'prayer warriors' to intercede for you. O.K.?"

"O.K."

That was several years ago. Not only is Kristi in a wonderful relationship with God, she is close to her loved ones and she is still here with us.

"Spontaneous remission," the doctors called it.

"Yes, certainly," we responded. "And we know who caused it."

9. Not Enough Power in the Ones Ministering

If being an instrument of grace can be likened to holding God with one hand and the sick person with the other, our usefulness as an instrument depends to some degree on our grasp of both God and the sick person. If through ego, condemnation, superiority or laziness, we do not care about people, we will have a "faulty connection" on that end. The power will not flow through us into them. If, on the other hand, our grasp of God is weak, little or no power will flow into us in the first place. The power shortage can exist for several reasons.

We are faithless. We do not think God really wants to heal people or use us to do it. What then are we doing in a ministry of healing? We have taken a God-centered ministry of power and turned it into human love and sympathy. Human love and sympathy are not wrong, but they are woefully short of the fullness of what God wants for people and what He can do through His yielded vessels. Note where Jesus laid the responsibility for the disciples' failure to cast the demon out of the epileptic boy. When the disciples asked Him, "Why could we not cast it out?" Jesus responded, "Because of *your* little faith" (Matthew 17:19–20, italics added). "I don't expect anything to happen," one man told me. "I pray with people because it comforts them." How inadequate! Jesus did not just comfort people in their illness; He healed them!

We are lazy. Spiritual growth demands work, sacrifice, surrender. Many are willing to follow Christ at a superficial level but hit a plateau when much else is demanded. Although God can, and often does, use us in spite of our inadequacies, the person God uses best, regularly and most powerfully is the one who takes time to work hard on spiritual growth. Think, if you need convincing, about your golf game (or your equivalent of it). While even a duffer can hit the occasional incredible shot, it is best described as a fluke. Those who do well consistently are those who work at their game. Or, to use a musical analogy, take this old joke: "Question: How do you get to Carnegie Hall? Answer: Practice."

We are proud. We think we can effect healing by our own willpower or by checking in with God occasionally. This is especially likely if we have been used by God previously to bring people to wholeness. After a while we start to think we're "good at healing" and forget we need His moment-by-moment empowering. There have been times in healing services when I noticed a drop-off in "results." I realized that while I had started the prayer time for others with abject dependence on God, as the service progressed (and especially as things were happening) I relied less on God and more on my experience, knowledge and stamina.

We are embarrassed. For many of us, speaking of the things of God is embarrassing, no matter how deeply we believe them. Or we forget that while Christianity is personal, it is not private. We must overcome this reticence lest our ministry become merely armchair psychology.

Those of us ministering healing need to acknowledge humbly that part of the problem may be ours and not the person's to whom we are ministering. Yet how often have we been to healing services in which people were told, "If you're not healed tonight, it's because you don't have enough faith"? That may well be true, as we will see shortly. But it may be true that the problem lies with the one(s) ministering.

No, we should not allow Satan to condemn us when we fall short, or be deeply distraught at every failure. Nor should we forget that God can provide other means for those people we are not able to help. But at the same time, we may need to confess that *we* have let people down. Our attitude should be that of my physician-wife: "Many people are depending on me. By God's grace I've got to do the best job I can."

10. No Perseverance

Most people have no difficulty understanding the need for a lengthy course of medical treatments, or going to an osteopath or chiropractor for several sessions until a muscular problem is resolved. But many people seem to believe that if immediate improvement is not registered after one session, healing through prayer is a waste of time. Nothing happens or seems to happen, so they give up.

Since some healings are gradual, and perhaps involve a variety of factors coming into play, perseverance is necessary. Don't give up! God is just beginning to work.

This is why a church healing ministry that concentrates only on the occasional big healing mission fails to bring healing to more than just a few people. Much better, in addition to such missions, is faithful, week-by-week ministry in Sunday worship services. The ongoing "cure of souls" through confession, counseling, spiritual direction, preaching, teaching, prayer, worship, the sacraments and intentional, specific prayer for healing yields great fruit in people's lives.

My experience has been that those who avail themselves regularly of all these aspects of spiritual growth find them also to be preventive medicine. (See chapter 14 for further details.) We know there is a connection between the state of our emotions, the condition of our spiritual lives and disease. As emotional and spiritual problems are nipped in the bud, or even prevented from budding, many of the diseases that might have occurred are prevented.

Just as sticking to a diet or hanging in there with exercise is as challenging as it is rewarding, so, too, is presenting ourselves regularly for ministry.

11. Negative Thinking or Not Enough Faith on the Part of the Person Needing Prayer

It is perhaps here that the greatest controversy about healing occurs. For some, "not enough faith" is an easy solution to the problem of not being healed. For others, the idea that God would withhold a blessing because of some lack on our part is inconsistent with their view of God.

In fact, the Scriptures (illustrated, of course, in human experience) present a picture that is more complex. Our Lord performed hundreds of healings. We see this reflected in such statements as "many followed him, and he healed them all" (Matthew 12:15; Luke 4:40). We have, however, specific information about slightly more than three dozen individuals healed by our Lord. These "case histories" present a wealth of information. (See Appendix 3.) From them we see the relationship of faith and healing. In short, we discover that sometimes faith (or its lack) is a key in healing. At other times faith does not seem to be a factor.

Let's look first at faith—or, more precisely, faith in Jesus to heal—as a factor on the part of the sick person.

On several occasions Jesus ministered in response to a person's faith. "According to your faith be it done to you," He said (Matthew 9:29; also see 9:22). On the negative side we read the sad notation, "And he did not do many mighty works there, because of their unbelief" (Matthew 13:58).

Why is faith so important? First, we know the value of a positive mental attitude. Two people can be suffering from the same illness, have the same bodily strength to recover, yet one dies and the other lives. Physicians often use the phrase "the patient's will to live" to describe that intangible yet real component in the recovery process that is akin to faith. Faith can, at the very least, be like the placebo (literally, from the Latin, "I will please") effect of some so-called medicines. A placebo has no medicinal value. It serves as a stimulus to summon up one's will to recover.

The placebo effect is one reason (the other being satanic counterfeits) why there are cures in all sorts of religious healing services, sane or wild, Christian or otherwise. We Christians need not make ourselves look foolish by denying either the reality or the value of such recoveries. It is obvious that sick persons have recovered and we should be glad they are better—though we might inform them, if possible, that beyond cure of what ails them, the greater blessing of wholeness is found only in Christ. We might also be able to warn them that certain non-Christian healing practices, though obviously effecting something good in the short run, can do damage down the road, whether to their wallets, their emotions or their spiritual lives.

But faith is much more than positive mental attitude. It is trust in the Lord—in who He is, what He does and what He wants to do for us. Faith does not mean just believing certain doctrines (although this is important, for Jesus said it is the truth that sets us free—John 8:32). *Faith is also trust.* Faith is entrusting ourselves, our hopes, our fears, our needs, our hurts to God and giving Him permission to work on them.

God is respectful of our personhood. He has given us free will to accept or reject Him. He allows the believer to turn various parts of his life over to Him or keep control over them himself. This is illustrated in the story of the rich young ruler. Jesus wanted him as a disciple but the man chose not to pay the price (Matthew 19:16–22). Although Jesus encouraged him and warned him of the consequences of not following Him, the choice was ultimately the man's. In Revelation 3:20 we see faith likened to Jesus standing outside a door knocking. If anyone opens the door, He will come in. Although He wants very much to be inside, where His love and blessings can be more greatly received, He will not break down the door.

Faith as applied to healing means, "Jesus, I give You permission to go to work on my life. Fix what is broken. Point out to me what I have to do, and show me where my sins are blocking what You want to do. I trust You to do Your part. Please teach and empower me to do mine."

Many people do not want Jesus to work on their aches and pains because they know instinctively that He will not deal just with surface problems but will go to root causes deep within. Thus, a choice: "If the only way Jesus will enter my life is as Lord, I would rather stay sick." This choice may be conscious or buried deep in the soul, but if we decide to keep Jesus outside—if not of our lives, then at least of our problems—we should not find it cruel for God to honor that choice.

Always remember: Faith is not an emotion. Nor is it something a few people are lucky enough to have while others do not. Nor is it the possession of those with a certain personality type. *Faith is firm, confident trust in God who has proven Himself trustworthy.*

How, then, is faith engendered?

We can ask God for faith. We can be like the man who said to Jesus, "I believe; help my unbelief!" (Mark 9:24). It is a request God delights to answer.

Faith also grows as we meditate on who God is, what He has done for others in the past and what He has done in our own lives. Isn't it true that confidence in people comes over time from our dealings with them? As we observe them in a variety of circumstances, we get to know them and whether they can be trusted. So, too, with God. As we pray—unless our prayers are rote recitation or merely a list of wants—we learn about Him. As we read Scripture and Christian biographies, we see in a variety of people, many like ourselves, how God works. As we recall what God has done for us in the past, we remember His love and provision.

One aid to this, one practiced by many of the great saints of God throughout Church history, is to keep a diary, a journal or what I call a "miracle notebook." Whenever our faith wavers in God's ability or desire to bless us and help meet our needs, we can turn to page after page of accounts how at various times, in various needs and in various ways God answered our prayers. The result? Firmer confidence—*faith*. As we thus focus on God we emulate the psalmist who said, "I will call to mind the deeds of the LORD; yea, I will remember thy wonders of old" (Psalm 77:11).

Michael Baughen (pronounced *bonn*), Bishop of Chester, England, says, "We don't have to have great faith in God. What we need is faith in God who is great." Jesus told us our faith needs only to be as a mustard seed, the tiniest seed in the garden (Matthew 13:31–32). But that seed, to grow, needs to be watered, fertilized and protected from predators. Our devotional lives, practiced regularly and devoutly, water the seeds of faith so they will be sufficient when we need them.

What about times when faith is not present in the person who is sick?

There are times when personal faith falters. Often it falters when we need it most. The devil has snatched it from us, the busyness of life has choked it out or the bad experiences we are going through have acted like hard soil to keep faith from sprouting (compare the parable of the seeds and soils Jesus told in Matthew 13). In times like these, it is so good to be part of a community of faith upon whom we can lean. While obviously we cannot presume upon this—if everyone were always leaning on everyone else, the whole pile would soon topple or the one or two whose faith remains strong would soon be exhausted—what a joy it is for the faith of others to help us!

Roughly half of the accounts of our Lord healing specific individuals illustrate the results of such vicarious faith. Jairus, by seeking out Jesus, exercised faith on behalf of his daughter (Mark 5:22–23). The centurion did the same on behalf of his servant (Luke 7:2–3). Four men acted on their faith by raising a roof and lowering their paralyzed friend into Jesus' presence (Mark 2:2–5). In each case, Jesus healed the hurting person in response to the faith *of others*.

As priestly people of God (1 Peter 2:5, 9; Revelation 1:6), we can intercede for others, taking them confidently by the hand to God's throne of grace (Hebrews 4:16). What a responsibility this is, but what a privilege!

While the sick person may not need faith to believe that anything good will happen, he must allow God to work. In other words, while the sick person does not necessarily need to have positive faith in Jesus for healing, he does need to cooperate, however passively. Active "negative faith"—refusing to let Jesus go to work or dismissing anything good that starts to happen—can serve as a distinct barrier to healing. To go back to the analogy of Revelation 3, if we are lacking in faith we do not necessarily have to be the one opening the door when Jesus knocks, but if we refuse to allow someone to open it for us, or if we order Jesus out once He has been let in, He will usually leave, taking His blessings with Him.

This is not out of anger or punishment, but out of respect for the freedom He has given us.

What about the role of emotions? If faith is confident trust in God, where do the emotions fit in? As with so many things in the Christian faith, a fine balance is the answer. We know how music, worship and a beautiful sunset can engender a religious encounter with God. No doctrinal content is imparted, but something powerful is experienced, often to the strengthening of our faith. Affective—that is, nonrational, noncognitive—learning is important.

Let's use music as an example. Music can soothe, as we see when the young David played the lyre for Saul (1 Samuel 16:23). Music can inspire. As God dwells in the praises of His people (Psalm 22:3), music can release faith or deepen it. I know someone who was healed physically at an organ concert I once gave. A simple worship service can cut through all the religiosity and bring us face to face with Jesus and His love. An ornate liturgy can let our spirits soar as we enter into the lofty transcendence of God's majesty. A service beside a lake can minister peace to us, as can a candlelight service. All these things can help faith.

A few words of caution. Any experience of God must be checked against the truths of Scripture. Just as not all spirits are of God (1 John 4:1), neither are all religious experiences.

Nor are all uses of emotion-filled services wise. Joseph Goebbels used martial music and pageantry to manipulate the German multitudes into a frenzied desire for war. I have been at services in which people have been worked into a froth. Some healings occurred, but they were generally transient ones. The persons seemed to be healed but a few days later, when the emotional rush subsided, the problems came back. Emotion is good when it enhances faith, but not when it manipulates the worshiper.

What about the phrase "Please heal me if it be Your will"? While at first glance this sounds like a good prayer, a humble waiting on God's sovereign will, it sows seeds of doubt.

God has amply demonstrated His desire to heal us in what His Word says and in what Jesus did. Although there may be exceptions, we should not center our theology in the exceptions but in the dominant teaching of Scripture: God wishes to heal. To pray *if* bespeaks a rejection of Scripture. It is no different from praying, "Lord, give me Your grace to keep the Ten Commandments, if it be Your will." Such a prayer undermines belief.

We must be careful, on the other hand, not to tell God exactly what to do, when and how. In the so-called "positive confession" theology, the believer does that. He is encouraged to stand on the promises of God. That is good, so far. Unfortunately, he is then encouraged to go on and make a positive confession: "I am being healed" or even "I am healed right now." Not to believe that or to give any regard to the still-existing symptoms of the problem is, according to followers of positive confession teaching, a faithless "claiming" of the problem.

A fuller discussion of the theological difficulties we should have with such teaching will have to wait until chapter 8. Suffice it to say for now that such a belief is not faith, but presumption.

If the prayer "Lord, heal me if it be Your will" is a prayer of doubt, and the assertion "I am healed right now" is a statement of presumption, where is the balance? I believe the best prayer we can offer for healing is something like this: "Lord, confident in both Your promise and Your example, I know You are on the side of health and of my being healed. I pray, then, heal me *in accordance with Your will.* I affirm Your loving power and powerful love and I leave the details up to You." This balanced prayer affirms confidently the fact that God wants to heal us while it honors His sovereignty in allowing Him to determine when and how.

So what should we conclude about the relationship between faith and healing?

1. Faith is confident trust in God who has proven trust-worthy.
2. Faith involves emotions but does not center on them.
3. Faith is not a product of manipulation. Rather, it is a gift of God for which we can pray, and it is strengthened as we meditate on who God is and what He has done—as recorded in Scripture, in our lives and in the lives of others.
4. Faith helps us be healed in the sense that it gives God permission to work in our lives.
5. As the priestly people of God, we can pray effectively for others, especially to help those whose faith is weak or nonexistent.
6. Not everyone need have faith in order to be healed, but those who deliberately set up barriers seriously diminish the likelihood of being blessed.
7. To avoid the extremes of doubt and presumption, the best attitude to express is, "Please heal me, Lord, *in accordance with Your will.*"

12. God's Kingdom Realized Only Partially on Earth Now

The birth, life, death and resurrection of Jesus Christ began, in a new and special way, the kingly rule of God on earth. It began then and is spreading now. The rule of Satan, the prince of demons and the prince of this world (Matthew 12:24; John 14:30), is being rolled back. Even a cursory glance at the world situation will remind us that the defeat of darkness and the establishment of light is not yet complete.

I use the term *kingly rule* rather than *Kingdom* because it is a better translation of the New Testament Greek, and because the word *Kingdom* implies a settled territory under the control of a particular ruler. The reality is quite different. As with many a country involved in civil war, people in the same community, even the same family, give allegiance to different leaders, and the final victory of one group over the other has not yet occurred. Those following the Lord and those following the evil one (included in this are spiritually blind "fellow travelers," the spiritually indifferent) are still caught up in the raging spiritual warfare (2 Corinthians 10:3–4; Ephesians 6:12). The beachhead of God has been established but the final victory has not been secured. We are living "between the times."

How, then, should we live and what should we expect in terms of the pervasiveness of God's healing?

Perhaps I can illustrate by a comparison with the latter days of the Second World War in Europe.[1] On June 6, 1944, when the invasion of Normandy established the beachhead in Europe, British Prime Minister Winston Churchill said, "The war is over." Churchill did not mean all fighting had stopped. He knew much fighting and dying still lay ahead. But he also knew that because the Allies were now established firmly in Northern Europe, and other Allied soldiers were working their way up through Italy, the outcome of the war was no longer in doubt. The only unknown was when. On May 8, 1945, V-E Day was celebrated. On that day the war in Europe was—literally—over, and the blessings of peace could be celebrated confidently.

What would a wise sergeant say to his soldier during that "in-between time" between June 6, 1944, and May 8, 1945? It would depend on the soldier's attitude. If the soldier was despondent, wearied from fighting, longing for a decent meal, a warm, dry bed and reunion with loved ones, his sergeant might say, "Chin up! The war rages on but victory is in sight." Sad to say, some soldiers gave up emotionally just as the war was concluding.

But if the soldier was cocky, presuming on the military successes just secured and running around foolishly, the sergeant might say, "Head down! The victory is in sight but the war rages on." Sad to say, some soldiers moving about without their helmets died just before V-E Day.

In the spring of *circa* 30 A.D., Jesus established the beach-head on earth. His cry was, "It is finished" (John 19:30). This, please note, was not an agonized cry of despair; He did not say, "*I* am finished," but, "*It* is finished"—the work of redemption. His atoning death on the cross marked the beginning of the end for Satan. Historically the Church has described this, variously, as our Lord's wrestling Satan and winning, though momentarily dying in the process (Colossians 2:15; see Gustav Aulen's book *Christus Victor* for a good expression of this understanding of the atonement); or as Jesus giving Himself as a ransom payment to free souls locked in Satan's prison (Mark 10:45; see Leon Morris' masterful exegesis of the word *ransom* in *Apostolic Preaching of the Cross*).

At some time in the future, a time Jesus said even He did not know (Matthew 24:36), He will return. His Second Coming will be the ultimate V-E Day, Victory-Earth Day, for at that time the kingdoms of this world will become the Kingdom of our God and of His Christ, and He shall reign forever (Revelation 11:15).

What might a pastor say to the Christian community as we now live between the times? To the despondent, to those believers burdened with their struggles against sin, the fiery darts of the enemy and recurrent sickness of body and soul, he would say: "Chin up! The victory is assured. We are no longer in darkness. Messiah has come. 'The people who walked in darkness have seen a great light' (Isaiah 9:2). 'Greater is He who is in you than he who is in the world'" (1 John 4:4, NASB).

But to the cocky, to those who, because Christ has come into their hearts, expect that all should be well, the battle against temptation easy, every prayer answered immediately and all sickness taken away quickly, he would say: "Head down! The battle is still on. We still wrestle against principalities and powers (Ephesians 6:12). We still succumb to sin. Some sickness still occurs, some even remains. So be sober, be vigilant. Your adversary the devil still prowls around like a lion seeking someone to devour" (see 1 Peter 5:8).

What does this have to do with the question of why some remain sick? Simply that for all our prayers and faith, for all our making use of the various means God has given us for our healing and ruling none of them out, some believers will still get sick and a few will even stay sick. (While the general health of believing Christians, especially those who believe in and pray for healing, will be better than that of the general populace,[2] and while Christians experience many remarkable healings when they do get sick, we are not immune from sickness, and for some the road to healing and wholeness is long and bumpy.) Sometimes it is because of a lack in the sick person or in the community of faith, but sometimes it is because sickness is still abroad in the world, because Satan is not yet totally conquered. Sometimes he wins a little victory in us. To use an analogy, we may have an umbrella to keep off most of the rain, but occasionally, especially in a driving rain, some water still sweeps around the side and gets us wet.

It is important to acknowledge (to retain balance) that we are living between the times. Some churches act as if the Messiah has not yet come. They *say* that Christ has come but they *act* as if the kingly rule of the Lord has not begun, and that the blessings of His kingly rule are not yet available. As a result, they have no confident expectation that healing will take place. Other churches act as if He has already returned. They *say* that the Second Coming is in the future, but they *act* as if all God's blessings occur now, unsullied by any lingering satanic action, unhindered by the desperate actions of the losing forces.

We can remind both groups that in Communion we have a powerful, effectual sacrament, the appetizer course to the Messianic banquet (the "Marriage Supper of the Lamb"), but God and His people have not yet sat down to that banquet (Revelation 19:9). We can remind them that while the teachings of Christ are known and the barrier between us and the Father has been rent in two (Matthew 27:51), we still know only in part and see through a glass darkly (1 Corinthians 13:12).

Wonderful healing blessings are available now, but to expect total healing now is as presumptuous as sitting prematurely at the heavenly banquet table, claiming to have complete understanding or imagining we know God perfectly.

Failure to grasp the significance of living between the times for Christian healing has serious consequences for the Church community. Churches that are like the despondent soldier do not offer healing, or if they do, it is with little encouragement, expectancy or seriousness. Parishioners miss out on blessings they might otherwise receive. Churches that are like the cocky soldier offer healing confidently and frequently, but woebetide those who are not healed! Something must be wrong with the person, they figure, or he would be healed.

While this is sometimes true, it is not always. Too many people are still sick whose faith is strong, whose sins are confessed and repented of and whose compliance with everything that makes for healing is strong. The result? On top of their sickness come the judgment and condemnation—however masked with politeness—of their fellow Christians. Another result: They have to live in denial of the problem, to others and perhaps even to themselves.

I met a woman once who was obviously physically sick, yet she said she was fine. When I commented that she did not *look* fine, she told me that in her church she had learned to say she was fine even when she was not. If she told them her problem, they would scold her for "claiming" her illness and accuse her of having some deep, unconfessed sin, a rebellious spirit, laziness about the things of God, or worse.

"Then how do people get others to pray for their real needs?" I asked her.

"They don't. Everyone has to present a happy face at all times."

Sooner or later that church will collapse. The question is, how many people will be seriously hurt, emotionally and spiritually, in the meantime?

Sometimes Christians deny the problem even to themselves. Being sick may challenge one's mistaken theology of how the so-called victorious Christian life is supposed to work. For some, this means that a supposedly mature Christian believer should no longer experience major problems or illnesses. To admit to an illness means that one is not mature or that one's theology is faulty. I know an internationally respected leader in the charismatic renewal movement who denied his illness up until the moment it killed him, for those very reasons. Yes, sometimes living in victory means that the Lord will take the problem away. At other times we are, as a hymn puts it, "victors in the midst of strife."

There is mystery here. We affirm gratefully the beautiful testimonies of healing from many people, yet wonder why the Rev. Canon David C. K. Watson, one of the leaders of renewal and healing in the Church of England, who followed all the "rules" of what one should do when falling sick, died in his early fifties of cancer. We can also cite the example of the early death of internationally known charismatic pastor Jamie Buckingham. There is much we can affirm, yet much we do not know. Let's celebrate the blessings of healing, remove the roadblocks that are observable and removable and live in the mystery that only in heaven will it all be explained.

Discussion Questions

1. Use one or two sentences to paraphrase the essence of each of the twelve reasons enumerated why some are not healed.

2. A respectable scholar, seeking a precise, linguistically correct definition of the biblical word *faith* as used in

the context of healing, declared it to be *chutzpah*. What do you think he was saying?

Experiment

Repeat the experiment at the end of chapter 1, but with a new "patient." Use new ideas from your study so far.

5

Sin, Sickness, Repentance, Healing

One of the reasons people get sick and one of the reasons they stay sick is sin. I am not saying that every time a person is sick, it is because God is punishing him or her.[1] What I am saying is that there is often a connection, a cause-and-effect relationship, between sin and sickness, between repentance and health.

We see this connection made in Scripture. We read in Mark 2 that the forgiveness of the paralyzed man led to his healing (verses 5–12). We discover our Lord's admonition to the man at the pool of Bethesda in John 5 that he should "sin no more, that nothing worse befall you" (verse 14). We find a connection in James 5 between the elders' healing ministry of prayer and anointing and the call to confession of sin (verses 14–16).

Why this connection between sin and sickness, between repentance and health? God has given us principles for living. These principles work. We find that just as those who build a machine are the ones who provide the soundest direction on running it, the principles that God gives us lead to happiness, wholeness and health, because God is the One who made us in the first place. As Jesus said, "The truth will make you free" (John 8:32). God has given us the free will to go against what He has told us, and when we do, we sin. When we disobey, we are not so much breaking God's laws as we are breaking ourselves or others against them. Or, to use another image, when we sin against God we remove ourselves from the place where the shower of divine blessings falls. God has promised us abundant blessings and new life (see, for example, John 10:10 and 2 Corinthians 5:17), but we cannot always experience the blessings of health when our spiritual laziness or deliberate disobedience removes us from the place God has chosen to put the blessings. God has not proven unfaithful; we have (see 2 Timothy 2:12–13). In short, when we sin God does not harm us; rather, we place a barrier between ourselves and God.

Let me give a few analogies from medicine. If we smoke four packs of cigarettes a day, we should not be surprised that we suffer from shortness of breath or develop lung cancer. If we are promiscuous, we should not be surprised if we contract a sexually transmitted disease. In both cases, the negative consequences to our health are self-inflicted. We were not made to live in those ways, and when we do, we bring on ourselves various kinds of sickness.

Or consider this analogy. When I bought my car, the manufacturer provided me with a book on how the car should be operated. Since it is my car, I can choose to operate it within those guidelines or in opposition to them. I can put maple syrup in the gas tank instead of the recommended 89-octane unleaded gasoline. If I do, the manufacturer has not harmed the car. I have!

The harm of sin can be seen in three kinds of relationships: with God, with others and with ourselves. Please remember: This division of sin into three categories, while useful for discussion, should not lead us to believe things are divided this neatly in life. Still, all sin is in some way sin against God, others and ourselves.

Sins Against God

The most fundamental sickness a person has is estrangement from God. God is holy and our rebellion against Him has placed a barrier between us (Isaiah 59:2). Ever since the sin of Adam, people have bumped up against this barrier that keeps them from enjoying perfect fellowship and a life free from difficulty. When Adam hid himself from God (Genesis 3:10), he demonstrated his awareness of how sullied his relationship with God had become. Adam's new propensity to sin and his instinctive urge to run away from God have been part of the human condition ever since. From Adam we have inherited spiritual estrangement and a desire to disobey. This is what theologians call original sin. To that inheritance we add our own individual sins.

The consequence of sinning, according to Scripture, is physical and spiritual death (Genesis 3:19; John 3:18; Romans 6:23). When confronted with this divinely issued death sentence, many of us want to protest that our sins "aren't that bad." Such a protest only gives us away. The truly holy person, the man or woman whose chief aim in life is to please God, is usually the one most aware of how much he or she is still fallen. To object that God does not know what He is doing in issuing this sentence against us is, in itself, a sign of how much we want to be in charge of our own lives and deny God that right. It is not against the prevailing standards of society that we compare our own behavior, but against God's will for us. As Jesus pointed out in the Sermon on the Mount, we might not be committing adultery literally, but anyone who lusts after another in his heart has, in God's eyes, committed that sin (Matthew 5:27–28).

Because God is holy, no sin is excused. We would certainly rail at God if the sins of mass murderers and rapists were excused. But if God were to grade on the curve, exactly where would the line be drawn? Sin has to be punished. And yet is there no hope? Because God is loving as well as holy, He opened a way that upholds both punishment of sin and for-giveness of the sinner.

I suppose God could have chosen many ways to do this. He did it by sending Someone to pay the penalty of our sins for us. Throughout the Old Testament we see God prepar-ing His people for that Person by instructing the Jews to sac-rifice unblemished lambs as offering for their sins. They came to see that sacrifice for sin is necessary, and that unless they were going to suffer the consequences themselves, they needed someone or something to do it for them. Year by year the sacrificial lambs were offered to prepare God's people for the coming of Jesus, the "Lamb of God, who takes away the sin of the world" (John 1:29). By offering Himself on the cross as a pure sacrifice for sin (Romans 5:8; 1 Peter 2:24; 3:18; 1 John 3:16), Jesus became the Savior of those who would put their trust in Him. Those who received Him were given forgiveness of sins and adoption as sons and daughters of God (John 1:12).

God's upholding of both His holiness and His love is the model the Church is to follow. Some churches, usually extremely conservative ones, uphold God's standards in such a way as to bring condemnation on those who fall. They not only hate the sin; they hate the sinner. The problem rampant in the mainline denominations is the opposite. In an attempt to be accepting and inclusive, they require no repentance but view any behavior as acceptable. They not only love the sin-ner; they love the sin.

We find New Testament balance in the way Jesus reached out to the woman caught in the act of adultery (John 8:3–11). While He refused to condemn the woman, He exhorted her not to sin again. The apostolic Church debated whether or not to include Gentiles (Acts 15). They concluded that Gen-tiles could be admitted, but only if they forsook pagan prac-tices. For the Church today to be true to the teaching and example of her Lord, we must demonstrate a similar "love-the-sinner-hate-the-sin" attitude. We are to reach out with love to those who are marginalized by society and call them (as the Lord calls everyone) to forsake their sin and turn to Him.

In addition to being the Savior of individuals, Jesus inaugurated the Kingdom of God. Although its completion comes at His Second Coming, we taste substantial fruits of it now. While emotional turmoil rages around us and within us, it is still possible on earth to enjoy the "peace of God, which passes all understanding" (Philippians 4:7). We may get sick, but healing is available. Our human bodies are subject to decay, but believers in Christ will rise to newness of life with Him.

As for this latter point, it is wrong, theologically and pastorally, to encourage someone by saying that in death God took a loved one home. Rather, *death* took the loved one from us, but for those who have put their trust in Christ, God has taken away death from that person.

How do we receive Christ's free gift of eternal life, this now-and-forever healing of the most fundamental of all sicknesses—estrangement from God? We receive it as we do any other gift: We simply take it with thanks. If you have never done this, or if you are not certain that Christ has taken the penalty for your sins, you might offer a simple prayer to God like this: "Heavenly Father, I admit to You that I am a sinner. I have sinned in thought, word, deed and by what I have failed to do. I acknowledge that I cannot earn my salvation but need Jesus to be my Savior. I know that He died on the cross to pay the penalty for my sins. I now ask Jesus to be my Savior, to take the penalty of my sins away so that I can have fellowship with You, both now and in heaven. Thank You, Jesus, for being my Savior. Amen."

When we receive Jesus as Savior, we also promise to receive Him as Lord of our lives. It is not possible to separate the two. No Christian believer will ever be free from committing sin. But what God wants when we ask Jesus to be our Lord and Savior is, first, our desire to surrender to Jesus as Lord, and second, a regular, good-faith effort to do our best, instructed by the Scriptures and aided by the Holy Spirit.

Even after a person has received Jesus as Lord and Savior, there can be spiritual sickness from time to time. To be sure, it is far less serious a problem than before he came to salvation. But it is a problem nonetheless. Suppose I were adopted into a family and had a fight with my adoptive father. I would still be his son but our relationship would be impaired.

The degree to which a Christian is aloof from or rebellious toward God is the degree to which the relationship with God is sick. God did not send Christ to die for our sins only to have us accept salvation but reject a personal relationship with Him. God made us to know Him, to enjoy Him, to give Him glory, to be beloved by Him and to live according to His commandments.

As for aloofness from God, we must remember that, while our good behavior is important, *God first wants us.* Let me give you an example.

When I was doing my graduate work in England, I stayed with a number of families during vacations. One was a working class family living in Birmingham. There was a lot of noise and confusion in the home, the children did not always do everything they should and harsh words were sometimes exchanged. Apparent immediately, though, was a deep and abiding love between children and parents. Another family with whom I stayed was upper class and lived in a posh section of London. There were wealth, luxury, even "hot and cold running servants." The children were polite. They observed all the social graces. They never seemed to do anything wrong. But it became obvious that their relationships with their parents were built on formal politeness, not love. Any love they had was for the nannies and governesses who reared them.

I have often asked parents which sort of children they would like. Nearly everyone opts for the children who, despite their faults, are in a relationship of closeness and warmth.

One woman added, "The behavior we can work on later." Is
God any different from this?

As for rebellion against God, spiritual sickness can also
come through slipping back into spiritual lethargy or by an
intentional refusal to make Jesus Christ sovereign over one's
life. The earliest creedal formula in the Church was the simple statement "Jesus is Lord" (1 Corinthians 12:3). Many
Christians are quite willing to worship God, do things for
God and ask favors of God. The stumblingblock is obedience. Jesus saw many who were, in effect, religious dilet-
tantes, following Him for whatever they could get out of it.
They did not want to obey. "Why do you call me 'Lord,
Lord,' and not do what I tell you?" He once asked (Luke
6:46). Our love of God, while of course involving thoughts
and emotions, includes much more. "If you love me," said
Jesus, "you will keep my commandments" (John 14:15).

Keeping the commandments—as our Lord pointed out to
the Pharisees—is much more than do's and don'ts (Matthew
23:23ff.). It far transcends the usual self-congratulatory feelings of virtue we bestow on ourselves for refraining from
murder, adultery or armed robbery. Fundamentally it is attitude or disposition. Do I want to do just what is societally
respectable, or is my fundamental desire to please God in my
innermost being by comparing every aspect of my thoughts,
words and deeds with His revealed will?

Community standards of what is acceptable have changed
considerably in the past few decades. Some etiquette writers
have revised their works to supply "proper" ways to do various things that God still rules out. Several etiquette books,
for example, now list the "correct" way to address a wedding
invitation to two people living together apart from marriage.
When I was growing up in a small Massachusetts town in the
1950s, it was possible to lean on community standards without a detailed knowledge of the Scriptures, because those
community standards were fairly close to God's will. This is
no longer possible. Apart from a careful examination of the

revealed will of God in Scripture, it is likely that we may be approved by others in polite society while breaking many of God's commandments.

Understood this way, we see why the Pharisees (for all their religious observance and squeaky-clean morality) and the rich young ruler (for all his rectitude) fell so far short. God wants more than believers; *He wants disciples.* We are to observe everything He taught (Matthew 28:20). To do less is sin.

In identifying our own sins for the purpose of amending our lives, I find it helpful to study Scripture with Christian believers who come from different cultural or political backgrounds. While I insist that they believe in the authority and reliability of Scripture as the Word of God (otherwise we are simply debating religious opinions, not standing under the revealed will of the Lord), it is helpful when they come from different backgrounds than my own. The reason for this is simple. No matter how committed we are to the Lord and to His written Word, no matter how much we ask the Holy Spirit to guide our understanding, we read the Bible with blinders on.

Several years ago I spent some time teaching clergy in various locations around Kenya. Toward the end of my stay in one location, I pulled aside the local bishop, a man I had known when he studied in Boston, and told him that while there was much admirable in the spiritual life of Kenyan Christians, I was puzzled about how these otherwise obedient disciples could be so unobservant of the Lord's clear teaching in certain matters.

"It's our cultural legacy from the days before we knew Jesus," he said. "In spite of a century of teaching, our people are still blind to what God's Word says about these things."

I was starting to feel satisfied until he continued, "When I studied in America, I noticed that while there was much that was admirable in the spiritual life of American Christians. . . ."

One of the ways we can overcome cultural blinders is by studying Scripture with believers from other cultures, with the understanding that we will set aside superficial politeness and lovingly hold one another accountable.

We can note the same blindness when it comes to ideology. Simply put, biblical Christians who are "conservative" by nature tend to be more attuned to some scriptural commandments than to others, while biblical Christians who are "liberal" by nature tend to do the same thing with different scriptural commands. Once again, the solution is the same: Study Scripture with people who uphold the authority and reliability of all of God's Word, but who come with different ideological makeups.

Sins Against Others

Such sins as resentment, bitterness, jealousy and unresolved anger hurt us spiritually, emotionally and physically. Let me give you an example. I was once teaching at a renewal conference at a church in New York. As I did not have to leave right away after the conference, the rector asked if I would accompany him to visit a sick parishioner—a woman bedridden with some paralysis. I was not in the woman's room for more than a minute before she launched into a stream of angry invective against her sister. She accused her of all manner of wickedness. I tried to suggest gently that God's will is forgiveness and that sometimes paralysis comes from our attitudes. (This was not anything original with me, nor was it particularly a Christian insight. Medical people of a variety of religious outlooks have said the same thing. Nor was it being judgmental on my part. It was simply a diagnosis of the situation.)

"I'd rather be bedridden than forgive that no-good sister of mine!" she shouted at me. I tried to tell her that that might be exactly what would happen.

I had occasion a year later to speak to her rector again. "Is So-and-So still angry?" I asked him.

"Yes," he replied.

"Is she still bedridden?"

"Of course."

Another year passed and I was invited back to the church to teach once again. I made sure I visited the woman.

"I suppose you're going to try to convince me to forgive my sister, aren't you?" was how she greeted me when I entered her room.

"No, actually, I'm not," I replied. My thought was that nothing short of a dramatic confrontation would get through, much as an intervention of tough love is sometimes the way to get the message across to an alcoholic. "Quite honestly, your attitude and health do not affect me one bit, except for the fact that I do care about you. You can be bitter; you can forgive. It's your choice, not mine."

After a very long pause, she looked at me through heavy eyes and said, "I'm tired of being bedridden. I'm tired of being angry. I know I should forgive, but how? I don't feel it even though I know I should."

Forgiveness, I told her, is not a matter of feelings. Forgiveness is a choice we make, and it involves several steps.

First, she should ask God for grace, for we cannot do this without His help.

Second, she should confess her own faults—not just the sin of bitterness, but every sin in her life she could remember. Part of the reason for this was to remind her that she was no better, sinwise, than her sister (see Matthew 7:5).

Third, she should pray blessings for her sister. Often when we "pray" for others, we are really telling God how to change them. It is an attitude of judging, of superiority—hardly the framework for forgiveness. Positive prayers are prayers that God will bless them, make things go well for them and so on. I have found it difficult to stay angry at someone for whom I am regularly praying positively. These prayers may at first be offered out of sheer duty, but eventually our feelings will mellow. The *feeling* of forgiveness follows the *action* of forgiveness.

Fourth, as these things were underway, she should start praying for reconciliation. One must be very careful to make sure the motive for this is correct. To call up someone, no matter how badly he or she treated us, and say, "I'm calling to tell you I have forgiven you for all the bad things you've done to me," is hardly going to effect reconciliation. A better attitude and approach is to say, "We've been estranged for some time now. I know that I've done and said things that have been wrong. I know I've hurt you. I ask your forgiveness."

Some people use the word *sorry* when asking forgiveness, as in "I'm sorry we had a fight." Sometimes all that does is express regret without actually admitting fault. While it is certainly unhealthy to wallow in guilt or blame oneself for everything, whether responsible or not, neither is it always enough just to say, "Sorry." Far better is to say, "I've been wrong; please forgive me."

Often something wonderful happens. Humbling ourselves and asking for forgiveness can release the other person to do the same. So many times in asking forgiveness I have been told, "Mark, I do forgive you. But part of the fault lies with me. Please forgive me for how I treated you." Not only does such reconciliation remove a barrier and reestablish a relationship; often the relationship is much stronger.

But a note of caution. Asking for forgiveness is not always met with a reciprocal request. Sometimes we hear, "Well, I should certainly hope so, after the way you behaved!" In cases like that we are not to say, "Wait a minute! I did my part; now it's your turn!" That would nullify the step of asking forgiveness. We would be building the wall of estrangement back up again. Even if only ten percent of the sin that led to the initial estrangement was our fault, we are responsible for that ten percent. We are not responsible for the other person's part. Let God deal with him or her on that.

There may be little else we can do about another's attitude except to pray. Realize, however, that feelings of anger may well up within us because of his refusal to be reconciled or to ask our forgiveness. These have to be dealt with. Otherwise, if repressed or denied, they will lead to bitterness and resentment.

Forgiving others does not mean that we have to allow inappropriate behavior to continue. Forgiving a spouse who beats you does not mean returning home for more. Forgiving an alcoholic family member does not mean continuing to cover for him or her. To make either of these responses, far from being an act of forgiveness, demonstrates the need for ministry to the one "forgiving" so inappropriately.

The spouse returning home for another beating may be evidencing a subconscious self-loathing attitude of "I'm a nobody and worthy only of more abuse." More appropriate is this response: "I will forgive and pray for you, but I will no longer submit to beatings. I will work on my own inadequacies and inform you that until you get serious, sustained help, I will not return to you." Making excuses for an alcoholic, far from being an act of Christian love, may be an expression of codependent "enabling." While we are to love the alcoholic and let go of any bitterness or judgment, we must let the alcoholic take responsibility for his or her behavior. Such "tough love" may be the only way the alcoholic will face the truth about his or her problem.

Just as we can sin against others, the sins of others can harm us. If an unscrupulous company dumps its toxic waste near a water supply, for instance, the local residents might become physically sick. Or if a person has been molested in his youth, he or she might grow up with various emotional disorders, some of which might cause physical illness. Here, too, is a critical factor in our search for healing. We will examine it more fully in the next chapter.

Sins Against Ourselves

Our bodies are the temples of the Holy Spirit (1 Corinthians 6:19). They do not belong to us, but are God's property.

We are called to be good stewards of them. If we harm them by wrong actions or by neglect, we are damaging what belongs to God, and we render ourselves less able to do His work. Here is yet another example of how sinning against ourselves is sinning against God and others. Under this heading of the stewardship of our bodies come exercise, the right amount of sleep, diet, weight, rest or playtime relative to work, and so on.

Unfortunately, in some Christian circles this has been expressed in a selective legalism against certain "taboos" while other harmful practices are not mentioned. I remember as a teenager hearing a fiery Pentecostal preacher rail away against tobacco and the harm to one's body it causes. My concern while listening to him, though, was whether this 300-pound man would make it through his sermon without suffering a heart attack! His harangue against the "demon weed of tobacco" was based not so much on a consistent theology of turning from that which could harm the body as it was on specific taboos in his denomination. He was right to sound a warning about the harmful effects of tobacco, but he should have been more comprehensive in his understanding of what harms us.

As good Christian stewards, therefore (as well as people concerned about our health), we need to examine carefully how we take care—or do not take care—of our bodies. Not to do so is sin, and it can hurt us.

Similarly, we sin against and harm ourselves by wrong attitudes. The stressed, hard-driving, impatient, anxious person is more likely to be ill. Jesus tells us, "Do not be anxious" (Matthew 6:25). While our Lord did not say, "Be irresponsible," He does want us to let the burden of the solution to things rest with Him. Long before the phrase *Stop and smell the roses* became popular, our blessed Lord invited us to "consider the lilies" (Matthew 6:28). He considered foolish the stress-producing—and therefore disease-producing—rat race to achieve and acquire (Matthew 6:25–33).

The body, via what medical people call the sympathetic nervous system, turns attitudes and emotions into chemicals, many of which can stress the physical body. As my father's doctor once told him, "Hedley, your ulcer is not what you are eating. Your ulcer is what's eating you." While continuing to be responsible, we are to cast our care on God who cares for us (1 Peter 5:7).

We are not talking here just about eating less red meat and more turkey, or taking an occasional extra day off, although these are not bad ideas. Rather, we are talking about a major reorientation of lifestyle, of values. No wonder Jesus described it as being "born anew" or "born again" (John 3:3). Jesus is not asking us merely to believe in Him. The evil spirits did that (James 2:19; Luke 4:34)! Nor is He asking us to become more "religious." The Pharisees were that, and more!

Rather, He is asking us to have a new way of life, one based on trust in and dependence on God, one of gentleness, of different goals and different means to those goals. No wonder the rich young ruler would not become a disciple. More than his riches needed to go. He needed to change his whole attitude about life (Mark 10:17–22). The cost is great, but eternity is at stake; and for many people, health is, too. Does it take a heart attack before you will reorder your life? Or, to use different imagery, do you have to be knocked flat on your back before you will look up?

Sin and Sickness: A Plea for Balance

To sum up, sometimes getting sick and staying sick is our own fault and sometimes it is the fault of others.

Another factor deserves mention, of course: Sometimes sickness is rooted in the activity of the evil one. The man born blind in John 9 was not blind because of any sin in his (or his parents') life. Job was certainly a godly man (Job 1:1), yet he was sorely afflicted. On occasion Jesus described an illness as being caused directly by Satan (Luke 13:16). My experience

confirms this. I have seen several people released from various physical, emotional and spiritual sicknesses as I ministered
deliverance to them. We will discuss this in more depth later.

In the matter of sin and sickness, biblical balance is sorely
needed. When sickness *is* our fault we need to take responsibility. Yet it is surprising how many people are ready to
attribute sickness to anything but sin. Why is this true in the
face of overwhelming biblical and medical evidence?

One reason is the confusion between affirming people and
agreeing with them. Many people confuse confrontation with
judging, condemning or rejecting a person. Since we are not
to stand in judgment of others, so this argument goes, we
must never imply that a person is in the wrong or in any way
responsible for his sickness. Isn't this belief farfetched? What
would you think if your physician tested your blood pressure
and refused to tell you how high it was for fear of being
deemed judgmental? Or if your physician thought to himself or herself, *My health isn't perfect either. Where do I get off
telling this person he has blood pressure problems?*

Some ways of presenting information *are* demeaning. Your
physician could say, "Are you ever a no-good reject! Just look
at that blood pressure!" Or, "God doesn't love people who
don't take any better care of themselves than you do!" To
speak in this manner would, of course, be wrong. But simply
to state that there is a problem with the blood pressure and
that something must be done about it is not. It is diagnostic
and necessary for treatment to begin. Of the same order is
informing people that certain behaviors or attitudes, which
are out of line with God's will as revealed in the Scriptures,
are sin and that they cause unwellness in body, soul and spirit.

In order to understand better the difference between
"tough love" confrontation of a person in sin, and judging
or condemning that person, consider the differences between
how God and Satan speak to us about our sin.

First, God speaks to us at appropriate moments, when we
are able to listen and to respond. He does not ruin every

moment of our day with a barrage of accusations. Satan, however, is a constant accuser. He will whisper insinuations at times when we can do nothing about the matter because we must focus our attention on the matter at hand.

Second, God speaks to us about only two kinds of sin: the sin we are in the midst of doing and those sins from the past not yet confessed. The purpose is our repentance. Satan, on the other hand, seldom points out present sin lest we turn from it. He often points out sins that we have already confessed and repented of, simply to make us feel miserable and defeated.

Third, God points out our sin as our Friend. Like a physician whose concern in discovering illness is that we be cured of it, God addresses our sin so that we can forsake it and return to Him. Satan points out our sin to make us either deny it or dwell on it. In either case, he directs us away from the truth and away from God, hiding in either denial or fear.

Fourth, God points out only those behaviors, attitudes and orientations that are against His will. Satan uses shame. God directs us to things that can and should be changed. Satan points out things that, while possibly embarrassing, are not sin, and over which we have no control. While God may say, "You *did* wrong," Satan will say, "You *are* wrong." He may also add, ". . . and stupid, and ugly."

Fifth, God directs to the future, toward hope. He reminds us that if we repent, He will forgive (1 John 1:9). He points out that even though some sins have temporal consequences that will never change, He will restore blessings to the penitent, though they may be different from what we threw away. Satan, meantime, is the purveyor of despair. "Nothing will ever change," he says. "You will always be like this. Why bother trying?"[2]

Another reason some people reject a connection between sickness and sin is that they refuse to believe in sin or in a God who sovereignly holds us accountable. Many people want to fashion in their own image a God who blesses us and agrees with everything we do, never asking us to change. What God calls sin they want to deem an "alternative lifestyle."

On the other extreme are those who assume that whenever one is hurting, it is one's own fault. Loud protests against this view are found in both the book of Job and Jesus' remarks concerning the man born blind. These people, in reaction to the overly permissive views just mentioned, wish so to uphold the holiness of God and humanity's accountability before Him that they go too far in the opposite direction.

Also, these people believe in a stern God. This view could be a projection of their own meanness. It might come from projecting onto God an image of fatherhood derived from unpleasant experiences with their earthly fathers. It might come from an overly strict religious upbringing. It might come from any manner of neuroses. In any case, their picture of God is One who punishes us for any slight infraction of the rules.

The balanced statement is found once again in James 5. Speaking about the interrelationship of sickness and sin, James exhorts the elders of the church to anoint the sick person for healing and pray for him and "*if* he has committed sins, he will be forgiven" (verse 15, italics added).

When someone falls sick or a sickness lingers, it is highly appropriate to ask whether sin is a causal factor. Remembering that sin occurs in what we do by thought, word, deed; in what we fail to do; that one sins against God, neighbor and oneself; and that sins run the gamut from unbalanced diet to gossip to adultery to bigotry; we should engage in a thorough examination of conscience, comparing ourselves against the standard of God's Word. The purpose of this is to indulge in neither self-condemnation or self-justification, but to discover where we are wrong, so that by God's grace we can confess our sins, receive His forgiveness and change our ways.

This change will always lead to greater health in our relationship with God because the estrangement between us, which sin causes, will be removed as sin is dealt with. This change will often lead, immediately or gradually, to greater emotional and physical health, since our bodies, souls and spirits all interconnect.

Confessing Our Sins to Another Person

Because of Jesus' atoning death on the cross, Christians have direct access to the throne of grace through Him (Ephesians 3:12). We can confess our sins to God directly and privately. We do not need anyone to mediate except Christ. Yet at times we can be greatly helped by others in the confession of our sins.

The book of James instructs us to confess our sins to one another (5:16). There are several good reasons for this.

We confess our sins to others to lead us to humility.

To confess our sins to another person forces us to be humble. We are sinners and have nowhere to hide. It is sometimes easier to confess to God than to another person because of embarrassment. It has been my experience more than once that I have refrained from some action I was contemplating because I knew I would be embarrassed later when I confessed it to someone. It was and remains an effective deterrent.

We confess our sins to others to remind us of the social nature of sin.

All sin, besides being against God, is against others. Nothing that we do leaves others unaffected—thus the folly of those who say that what they do behind closed doors or with a consenting adult is no one's business but their own. Suppose someone is so busy acquiring material goods that he has time for little else. He has sinned against those in his family, immediate and distant, who need his presence, attention, aid, counsel or nurture. Or suppose someone on the healing team is hung over from too much partying and his spiritual antennae are somewhat fogged. He may go through the motions of praying for the sick on Sunday morning—if he shows up at church at all—but will he hear God clearly should God direct him in a certain way, and will he be as effective an instrument of God's grace? To confess our sins to another person reminds us how our sins—all of them—affect others. Remember the wise words of John Donne, the seventeenth-century poet: "No man is an Iland, intire of itselfe."

Remember, if we have wronged specific people, we must ask their forgiveness and make amends to them, if possible, unless to do so would harm them further.

We confess our sins to others to keep us from being too hard on ourselves.

Many people are far too hard on themselves because of an overly strict upbringing, or a neurotic bent to their psyche, or lack of sound biblical instruction, or the insinuations of Satan whom Scripture calls the "accuser of our brethren" (Revelation 12:10). They deem something a sin when it may be, at worst, a matter of questionable taste, a breach of etiquette, a lapse in decorum or failure to observe an arbitrary custom. Or, if the matter *is* a sin, they confess it over and over again, not knowing that Jesus is the perfect sacrificial offering for our sins (1 John 2:1–2). They need to be reminded that to confess a sin to Him means that sin is put as far away from us as the east is from the west (Psalm 103:12), and that God has truly and lastingly forgiven us. What a wonderful opportunity there is in confession for someone wise in insights into human nature and armed with the good news of the Gospel to assure such people of their forgiven state and good standing with God!

We confess our sins to others to keep us from being too easy on ourselves.

Sometimes people are not remorseful enough. They fail to see how serious a matter sin is. Sometimes they, by their upbringing, have a convoluted list of sins that emphasizes trivialities or taboos of human devising and ignores graver matters (see Jesus' rebuke of the Pharisees for just this in Matthew 23:23). I know of a few churches in which a parishioner can be expelled for smoking but not for bigotry. I know some church folk who will go into a tirade if others do not use their brand of "inclusive language" but not mind one bit sexual relations outside the covenant of marriage. Sin is what God's Word says is sin. Often we need someone else to call us back to that standard.

We confess our sins to others to get spiritual guidance. The word *repent* means much more than sorrow or remorse. It means "to change direction, to amend one's life" (see Acts 3:19, for example). God does not want us to keep stumbling over and over with the same sins; rather, He wants us to become different people. True change takes place, of course, only by the grace of God. The fruit of the Spirit (Galatians 5:22–23) is exactly that: characteristics produced by the working of the Spirit within us. Yet we have our part to play. While only God can grow the fruit, you and I have a gardener's responsibility to tend the plants that produce the fruit. We have our duties in prayer, reading the Bible, worship, listening to God's voice and so on. Other people are helpful in this process of spiritual growth. Sometimes the person who can best help us by hearing our confession is not the one who would make the best spiritual director. Still, that person, as confessor, will have a guiding role in our lives.

I do not mean, of course, that such a person should run our lives to get us into servile bondage to them. Some in the so-called shepherding/discipleship movement of the 1970s went to excess here by requiring people to get permission—literally—before they remodeled the house, took a new job, moved away or got engaged. I *do* mean someone who can help us in our spiritual growth, both keeping us within the boundaries of orthodoxy and, within those boundaries, helping us find the style that is best for us; someone who can answer questions about our spiritual journey and give us wisdom from Scripture and personal experiences of walking with God.

We confess our sins to others so they can pray with us.

Not coincidentally, right after James exhorts us to confess our sins to one another, he reminds us that the "prayer of a righteous man has great power in its effects" (James 5:16). Through prayer God can show us our sins and the way to live a more holy life. Through prayer we can open ourselves to God to receive His power to change.

The scriptural injunction to confess our sins to one another needs to be heeded much more than it is. There are several reasons why it isn't:

Pride. We just do not want to admit to others that we have failed or done bad things.

Fear. We are afraid of rejection by those to whom we confess, perhaps because our lifetime experiences have prepared us for condemnation, ridicule or rejection.

Hypocrisy. The various difficulties a few well-known church leaders have gotten themselves into have left a bad taste in the mouths of many people toward religious leadership in general. As one man asked me, "Why should I confess to hypocrites?"

Prejudice. Some resist confessing their sins to others because of prejudice against the Roman Catholic Church. Confession sounds "Catholic" and some people assume that if something is done by the Roman Catholic Church, it must be wrong. (Ironically, in the matter of confessing sins to others, the Roman Catholic Church is far more biblical than many of those churches that proclaim themselves to be Bible-based.)

Negative experience. Many who have tried confessing their sins to other people have stopped doing so because for them it was not a particularly helpful experience. In some cases their confessors were of no help. In other cases their confessors breached confidentiality. Another way some people have experienced this ministry negatively is through a misuse of church discipline. Scripture tells churches to discipline the flock (see, for example, Matthew 18:15–17; 1 Corinthians 5; 1 Timothy 1:19–20; 5:20), but if it is carried out in an unloving, self-righteous way, we may turn from church discipline altogether.[3]

It is true that confession of sins to another person can be done in a wrong way. But *when done right,* when done sensitively, discreetly and biblically, confession to another person can be an occasion of great spiritual help, and of spiritual, emotional and physical healing.

Father Michael Scanlan, president of the University of Steubenville, Ohio, found that as he took hearing confession seriously, some people were being healed of physical ailments right there in the confessional. Should we be surprised that to confess and forsake one's sins can lead to physical healing, sometimes dramatically and instantaneously?

Who Is a Good Confessor?

We know instinctively we should not confess our sins indiscriminately. The question is, therefore, To whom should we confess? What do we look for in a good confessor? (These criteria can be applied, additionally, to people doing other kinds of ministry, such as pastoral counseling, spiritual direction, inner healing and so on.) We look for:

Godliness

Those to whom we confess our sins should have an active, growing, personal relationship with Jesus Christ as Lord and Savior. They should acknowledge sacred Scripture as the written Word of God and as the final arbiter in matters of faith and morals. Their lifestyles—public and private—should be consistent with profession of this faith. No, we are not to expect perfection from them or anyone else. All of us, even the most godly, will fall short. What we are to expect is a high degree of godliness on the part of our confessors, as well as their regular, intentional effort to grow into deeper spiritual maturity. Were any of these things not so, any advice they gave would not be "wisdom from above" (James 3:17). As Scripture puts it, there is a way that seems right, but whose end is destruction (Proverbs 16:25). We want God's ways.

Good listening

It is important not to butt in too soon with an answer or with advice, but rather to let the person confessing "get it all out." For our confessors to respond too quickly may short-circuit the important purging and cleansing process before it is complete. Listening also needs to be active listening—that is, looking for clues as to underlying patterns, so that these, and not just the surface symptoms, can be addressed.

Discretion

We would obviously be loath to share intimate details with someone likely to spread it around town or throw it up in our faces at a later time. Rather, we want someone who is close-mouthed and will not share with anyone without first securing our permission.

A note of warning, however. While the courts have upheld doctor/patient, lawyer/client and clergy/penitent confidentiality, such protection does not extend to a layperson's ministry of hearing another's confession. If someone begins to confess a crime to a layperson, therefore, the layperson should immediately warn this person that he might wish, rather, to confess to a priest or minister. A layperson can be compelled to testify in a court case. In some cases, possessing information about a crime and not reporting it makes a lay confessor an "accomplice after the fact."

Empathy

Empathy has been defined as "engaged enough to care, detached enough to guide." An empathetic person, in other words, truly cares, yet retains objectivity. We would not find helpful someone obviously just going through the motions or playing a role, someone unconcerned about us as an individual. Someone caught up personally in our life, on the other hand, might lose objectivity and excuse behavior that needs changing. We want that Pauline ideal of "truth in love" (Ephesians 4:15). We want the response that our life warrants, not cold professionalism or sentimental indulgence.

Wisdom

We want a confessor who knows more than the truths of the Gospel. We want someone who knows how to apply these truths to our situation. We want someone who has personally tasted the degradation of sin and the joys of sins forgiven; someone who knows the ways the devil tempts, the Lord forgives and the Holy Spirit sanctifies; someone who knows when we are feeling guilty because of actual, true guilt or because of neuroses or the accusations of Satan; someone who can help us understand when we are experiencing consolation and desolation in their true and counterfeit versions; someone who can help us on the pilgrim's way to wholeness.

Because of the importance of this ministry to people's wholeness, we need to encourage our clergy to become involved or more involved in the ministry of hearing confession. Too often our clergy are so distracted by the administrative details of running a church that they devote insufficient time to pastoring the flock.

We also need to recognize that certain laypeople can fulfill the role of hearing confession, albeit in a nonsacramental way. People with the characteristics of a confessor are present in most churches. In a few they are already at work offering their ministry to burdened people. In most churches, however, they need to be discovered, recruited, trained, deployed and supervised. It takes work to do this, but the benefit from these people, in their own kind of healing ministry, is well worth the trouble.

Sin and sickness. Repentance and healing. As we realign our actions and attitudes with God's principles, we will be more likely to move back under that shower of divine blessings God has planned for us—blessings no doubt evident in good health.

Discussion Questions

1. How is brokenness inherent in the human condition?
2. How is brokenness the result of sins against God?
3. How is brokenness the result of sins against others?
4. How is brokenness the result of sins against self?
5. How is brokenness the result of spiritual oppression?
6. What is the scriptural authority for confessing sins to God? What are the benefits of it?
7. What is the scriptural authority for confessing sins to others? What are the benefits of it?
8. Assess your own competence as a hearer of confessions.

6

The Healing
of Memories

We all carry memories that still cause pain, immature behavior and physical, emotional and spiritual sickness. We find ourselves unable to do certain things, unable to relate to certain groups of people or unable to go to certain places because of associations with painful experiences in our past. We find our emotions and reactions of today misshapen by harm done to us in the past, by things we did wrong in the past or both. We are blocked, in certain aspects of our lives or straight across the board, from becoming the happy, fulfilled persons we want to be and God wants us to be. The healing of memories is a chance to go back and reclaim the past, not changing it, but changing its influence on our lives. It is a chance to be released from the shame, guilt and pain that have hurt us for years and continue to affect us today.

We have all been exhorted to "shape up." While sometimes such a "tough love" exhortation is exactly what we need, other times it is cruel and useless. We would change if we could, but something is holding us back. I knew a woman, for example, who simply could not get on a bus. Everyone either teased or ridiculed her for this. In response, she tried harder and harder but could not get past the first step in the doorway without breaking out in a cold sweat and feeling faint. In counseling we discovered the reason: She had been assaulted on a bus years before. Though she was not consciously aware of that event in her past, the mere presence of a bus triggered an emotional crisis in her. The healing of memories set her free.

The healing of memories is not to be used as an excuse to continue wrong or harmful behavior. On the contrary, when we discover why we do what we do, we can deal with the causes and become more mature and responsible.

People often ask, "How can you change the past?" In one sense we cannot. We cannot, for example, remove the fact that that woman had been assaulted on a bus. What we *can* do is remove the present-day harmful consequences of it. As we give over to God any pain, shame or guilt from past experiences, we find ourselves freer to live happily today.

Scriptural Example

A scriptural example of the healing of memories is found in the life of the apostle Peter. Peter, when he stood beside a charcoal fire, denied Jesus three times (John 18:18–27). After the resurrection Jesus gave Peter three chances to be restored to fellowship with his Lord—beside a charcoal fire (John 21:9–17). I believe that, far from being a coincidence, the fact that Jesus encouraged Peter to express his love and that He did it beside a charcoal fire shows His deep insight into human nature.

For Jesus simply to appear to Peter and forgive him might be enough on one level. Relationally Peter would be back in fellowship with his Lord. Intellectually Peter would know he was forgiven. But emotionally Peter might not *feel* forgiven—something that would hinder his future ministry. Additionally, might there not be some vague sense of unworthiness, triggered subconsciously by the sight, smell or sound of charcoal fires through the years? Jesus, knowing this truth about human nature centuries before it was identified by psychologists, sought to rescue Peter and his future ministry from repeated experiences of shame and self-accusation whenever Peter was around a charcoal fire.

Contemporary Examples

Let's take a look at some contemporary examples.

I recall meeting a woman at a social function. We had chatted for only a minute when I became aware of feelings of anger rising up in me toward her. She had done nothing to make me angry. In fact, she was complimenting me on a talk she once heard me give! Nevertheless, I was feeling a good deal of anger toward her. It dawned on me what was going on. She was wearing a certain kind of perfume, the kind worn by a woman who, a few years previously, had done me a great deal of harm. Obviously I had not dealt adequately with either the hurts that woman had caused me or my sinful attitudes in response. Both the hurts and the anger had lain dormant subconsciously until triggered by the perfume at the social function. I sought, and received, healing for the hurts the woman had caused me. I confessed to God my sinful attitudes in response to them.

I wonder how many of our irrational fears, prejudices and bad behaviors are expressive of hurts in our past.

In addition to bad feelings and altered behaviors, sometimes physical illness can be traced to events of the past. I know a man who always seemed to come down with physical problems around the Christmas holidays. The pains were real. The sicknesses showed up on tests administered by his doctor. Yet many wondered why they always manifested around the end of December. Eventually we found out. He came from a large family and felt neglected by his parents. One Christmas as a child he came down with chicken pox.

All of a sudden he was the center of attention. Family members fussed over him. They went out of their way to make up for events he could not attend. It was his best Christmas ever! Although he did not consciously try to become ill at Christmas, something in his subconscious sent messages to his body that it would be a good idea to be sick, and his body responded accordingly. When we discovered this, we went to work on his lifelong feelings of inadequacy and insecurity. It was a long process of emotional healing for him, but it worked. He now has a happy Christmas each year without becoming ill.

Sometimes the hurts of the past keep us from functioning as we would like. I know a man who for years in his marriage found it emotionally difficult to be sexually intimate with his wife. He loved her and she was good to him. But sometimes even the thought of an embrace was enough to make him tremble. In counseling he was finally able to recollect the painful memories of having been sexually molested as a young boy. Though occurring many years before and in a very different context, those experiences were significantly altering his relationship with his wife.

Discovering the Root of the Problem

It is often important to discover the root or roots of the emotional and physical problems we face. Otherwise, despite all our hard work and best intentions, we may do nothing more than try to rid our lawns of dandelions by mowing off their tops. The visible manifestation may be removed, but the roots are still there ready to blossom forth once again in similar or different ways. How do we discover those roots? How do we identify those places where we need healing of memories?

First, we list the hurtful experiences from the past that come to mind quickly, memories that still hold considerable pain. We all know the expression "Someday we'll laugh about this." If, despite the years, we cannot laugh at certain bad experiences of our past, if we cannot recall them without emotional distress, then we need healing of memories. There are events about which we will never laugh, like assault, rape, divorce or the death of a loved one. The best we can hope for here is to be able to recollect the event without emotional pain. If thinking about them still causes great emotional distress, then we need a healing of memories.

Second, we examine those categories—such as place, time of the year, type of person or kind of event—in which fear or prejudice exists. I knew a woman who could not go into drugstores. Even the thought of it made her anxious. We found it was because she had been in a drugstore once when another woman had had a heart attack and died right next to her. Entering a drugstore triggered all the emotions of that event, emotions that had not adequately been dealt with. While she had forgotten *why* drugstores caused her such a problem, they nevertheless did. We worked backward from the problem to discover the cause and then forward to find the solution.

In terms of types of persons, I counseled a man whose instant, gut-level reaction was to run whenever he saw someone in uniform. The root cause of this was his watching, as a very young boy, a number of movies depicting soldiers butchering civilians. Until he was healed of this memory, his fear was that anyone in a uniform—even a letter carrier—was possibly going to harm him. Although he could not explain the reason for his fear, it was real and controlled his life.

Sometimes our fears or prejudices can be secondhand. Everyone knows people who fear or hate certain groups, not because representatives of those groups have done them harm, but because other people have instilled the fear or prejudice about them. If one grows up hating, say, the Irish, because of the bigotry of a family member, those messages need to be discovered and erased from our "memory banks" in order for us to be free.

Third, in order to identify where we need healing of memories, we notice those areas in which there is an inordinate or unrealistic attraction. Many people marry individuals because they remind them of someone else whom they admire. I knew a man who married a woman simply because she looked like the kindly teacher who befriended him in the sixth grade when bullies were picking on him. Even though his wife's personality traits were nothing like those of his kindly teacher, subconsciously he made the comparison based on physical appearance.

Fourth, we look at those areas of "inability" in which the inability is more of an emotional block than simply a lack of skill or interest. For example, I don't work on my car. Although I can do minor repairs in an emergency, I know little about auto repair and am not particularly interested in advancing the learning curve! I know a man, however, for whom the attempt to work on his car precipitates a severe emotional crisis. It began when, as a boy, he was helping his older brothers and their friends fix an old jalopy in their garage. In his inexperience, he broke a spark plug while trying to insert it. The other boys yelled at him and called him names, and he ran into the house, tears streaming down his face. From that day on he formed an emotional block to auto repairs. No one would think it odd just because auto repair is not an interest of his. Nor would anyone deem it a problem just because he is not good at mechanical things. But the fact that he gets emotionally distraught when a friend asks him to look under the hood of a car indicates that the healing of memories is needed.

Let's look at another example in which inability to function in a certain way is traceable to emotional distress in one's earlier years. I know a woman, whom I'll call Irene, who struck me as brilliant, yet held an unchallenging, low-paying job. When I told her it seemed to me that a woman with her abilities could have a leadership position and a high salary, she responded that she was not good enough for anything like that. I tried to convince her that several others agreed with me but she refused to believe it.

Over a period of time, through prayer and counseling, through encouraging her to think back to events in her formative years, and through asking her family for their insights, we discovered that in junior high school a teacher who disliked Irene had told her she was a C student and would probably not amount to much. That teacher was respected and his views carried weight. Somehow the message was internalized. It was as if Irene adopted a script for life written by this teacher. Throughout her life she had been subconsciously acting her part—that of a C student who would never amount to much. Not coincidentally, she had been an *A/B* student up until that point.

Until we uncovered the incident with her teacher, no amount of pointing out the facts made a difference. Once we discovered the "taped message," as it were (deeply imprinted on her subconscious), erased it and recorded a message reflective of the facts, Irene gained confidence and fulfilled her God-given potential.

Fifth, we ask others for their input. They may know certain details of our lives that we have forgotten or repressed. They will often be able to point out behaviors we do not see in ourselves.

As for forgotten details, I know one man, whom I will call Sam, who was terribly afraid of dogs. Every time he saw one, his heart started racing. He could not figure out why. He knew of no unpleasant experience with a dog and he liked all other kinds of animals. Sam knew himself well enough to know it was far more than just preference, it was fear! We prayed together on several occasions to see if God might show us what the root of the problem was, but nothing came to us.

One day Sam called me.

"I know the source of the problem," he said. "I asked my aunt if there was an incident in my childhood that might have led to my fear of dogs. 'Oh, yes,' she said. 'Don't you remember the time when you were three and that Great Dane chased your tricycle, knocked you over and bit you on the leg? You've been afraid of dogs ever since. Don't you remember that?'"

The root problem in hand, we could proceed with inner healing. Dogs are not his favorite pet today (he prefers gerbils), but the fear is broken.

Our friends can also point out behaviors that may have hindered us all of our lives, but of which we are unaware. Tim had a certain pattern of behavior in dealing with people. Try as he might he could not figure it out or get a handle on what was causing it. A job relocation brought Tim into contact with a new group of colleagues, one of whom observed that he had all the behavioral symptoms of an adult child of an alcoholic parent. Instantly the lights went on. He *was* the adult child of an alcoholic parent. The colleague lent him some books on the subject. Now prayers, efforts and ministry had a specific focus. The enemy, previously elusive, was out in the open, recognized and more easily defeatable.

Sixth, we can flush to the surface past memories—good ones as well as bad ones—by picking a year in our lives and recollecting as much about it as we can. We make, as it were, a collage, full of items appertaining to that year. As we construct this collage, we will find all sorts of memories, long forgotten, coming to conscious thought.

Into this collage (either a work of art or a mental picture) go photos of ourselves, family and friends; headlines of significant news stories; songs that were "top of the pops" that we heard many times; images of what our home, neighborhood, school and church looked like; recollections of what was "in" fashion-wise; pictures of the cars of the era (the advertising pages of old *Time* or *Life* or *National Geographic* magazines are helpful here); items from diaries or scrapbooks or old letters we might have saved; any instances of significant events that we can remember; and so on. The more the better.

Every time I pick a year in my life to make a collage, three kinds of memories come to me. The first are pleasant memories. Recently I remembered with fondness a trip I took with my grandfather. These memories are for celebrating. Second are memories of unpleasant things that no longer cause emotional pain when I think about them. These events were not pleasant at the time, but at least they no longer cause emotional distress or negatively affect my life. These memories do not need healing.

Third, however, are memories that, to recollect them even years later, *do* make me upset. When I examine them, it becomes apparent that they control me in some way. These memories are grist for the mill of the healing of memories.

Which year do you start with? It depends. You might want to start with a year known to be generally happy so as to learn how to get in touch with the past by starting with something pleasurable. Or you might wish to focus on a year known to be problematic, so as to get right to the heart of the distress immediately.

The **seventh** and last way we identify those places where we need healing of memories is by asking God to reveal to us what might be wrong. Through dreams and visions, through words of knowledge (1 Corinthians 12:8), through the "still, small voice" with which God sometimes speaks to us (1 Kings 19:12), He can show us not only problem areas in our lives, but also their root causes.

A friend of mine asked God why she was standoffish to a particular uncle of hers. He always seemed friendly to her and everybody liked him, but the block remained. One day while praying, she got a picture of a small girl who looked like herself and a man looking very much like a younger version of her uncle. She saw the man trying to take something away from the child while she tried desperately to hang onto it. Finally, with a mighty tug, he wrested control of it from her. With that she went running off, crying her eyes out. "You know," she told me, "that must have been the incident that triggered the bad feelings I've had for him all my life." After a minute's pause, she added, "How foolish! In the pictures that came to me while praying, I saw what he was trying to take from me: a can of toxic chemicals!"

It is important not to try to gather all the information of painful memories at one time. If we were to spend a concentrated effort accumulating in our conscious thinking all the hurts of our earlier years, we would most likely be so overwhelmed as to become seriously depressed or even suicidal. Rather, we should work on one or two problems from the past at a time, either to their solutions or until it seems wise to leave them and go on to another one.

Dealing with Unpleasant Memories

Some painful memories are easily dealt with. Others require more attention. Here is a progression of steps that can be followed to minister the healing of memories, starting with the easiest.

1. Allow the problem to be brought to mind.

Often we are affected by an event of the past buried in the subconscious. We fight thinking about it, not wishing to relive the bad experience, feel the shame or pain again or do the hard work of overcoming it. Yet sometimes our simply allowing ourselves to become aware of the bad event is sufficient to break its power over us. Sometimes, however, that is not enough.

2. Talk about it with others.

Sharing an unpleasant memory with a trusted friend, a member of the clergy, a prayer or support group or a professional counselor will bring healing. This is one of the reasons for the popularity of groups like Alcoholics Anonymous. We discover we are not alone; others have similar problems. We can share our problems with them without fear of ridicule and in so doing place the problem out in the open where it can be dealt with. In some cases we discover that the problem, when it is out in plain view, is not as enormous as we once thought when we had kept it hidden. Sometimes we discover that others with similar problems have learned to cope well, or have been able to find freedom from the damage of the past.

Although it may be sufficient just to share the painful experience, sometimes it helps to hear affirming truths about ourselves. This is especially useful if our emotional pain comes from the lies of others. Sometimes this cathartic role can be played by trusted and trustworthy friends. Although they probably will not have had the same hurtful experiences we have, they will nevertheless accept us lovingly and let us talk things out. The kind of person in whom we confide should share similar characteristics with the person to whom we confess our sins. (Review pp. 103–105 for the description of who makes a good confessor.) A number of therapists have told me that at least fifty percent of their clients do not need professional help. They could find considerable healing by talking with a good friend in whom they confide. Sad to say, many people lack even one such friend.

There are times when we are just too afraid to share with a friend, or our friends are loving and supportive but too prone to give immediate advice without letting us get the problem out. In these instances a therapist or member of the clergy might be most helpful. With their training and experience they will, in many cases, be the affirming presence and listening ear we need. Many people find, particularly with those memories that hold a great deal of shame and guilt, that a counselor or member of the clergy not previously known to them is the best choice. I have counseled people whom I was not likely to see at a church function or at the Communion rail. Thus they felt freer to be more candid and relaxed than they would have been with their own ministers.

3. Pray for healing.

Sometimes simply talking it out is sufficient to get a person free. But many times the problem still persists. Thank God we have a rich resource for healing in prayer! Why is prayer so helpful?

First, because in prayer we open the door for the Lord to enter into our problems (see Revelation 3:20). So often God, who wishes very much to help us, waits for our request. As I mentioned before, this is because He respects our free will, given to us by Him in the first place. He did not make us robots. He will not treat us like robots now. In addition, if we are not ready to ask for His help, we are probably not able to receive it should it come. James' observation is relevant: "Ye have not, because ye ask not" (James 4:2, KJV).

Second, prayer is important because God knows us better than we know ourselves. He knows our problems and their sources. In prayer we let the Master Diagnostician go to work.

Third, prayer is important because God has the power to effect change. I have heard repeated observations about secular therapists being good at finding out the problem but not as good at solving it. God's power, made available to us as we pray, can transform our memories, removing their harmful effects.

Our praying need not be elaborate or fancy. Sometimes all we need in order to be healed is a simple prayer like this: "Lord Jesus Christ, I am frightened of flying since my friend was killed in a plane crash. Please take this fear away. Amen." Or the prayer may be one of surrender: "Lord, I yield to You these painful and unhappy memories of being beaten by my father. Please cleanse them and make me whole. In Jesus' name. Amen."

Sometimes, however, we need to pray at some length for the healing to get to the depths of a wounded soul. Dr. Francis MacNutt has popularized the phrase *soaking prayer* to describe how healing prayer sometimes needs to soak in over a period of time.

In some instances we can minister inner healing through prayer by ourselves. At other times, we need the prayers of others.

Fourth, prayer is important because God is love. Many are reluctant to relive painful memories. Yet as God goes to the root of the problem, He also comforts us. The pain involved in the healing process is much more bearable because He walks the road to wholeness with us.

In prayer we offer the Lord our hurts, fears, anxieties—whatever seems to be harming us—and ask for His help. It may come instantly or gradually. God might show us the root cause or heal the problem without our ever knowing what started it. He might heal us sovereignly while we remain mostly passive in the process, or He might tell us something we need to do. We should not expect every session of prayer for the healing of memories to be alike. The crucial things to remember are that God wants us made whole, that He is both the source of our blessings and the goal for our lives and that we need to listen to what He is saying to us every step of the way.

4. Receive holy Communion.

In Communion we have what Bishop Serapion, a bishop in the early days of the Church, called "specific medicine for our souls." As we receive Communion we lay our burdens, sins and hurts at the foot of the cross and receive grace to be made more whole. While this often comes when we are not thinking specifically about His grace, we discover that when we lay our burdens at the Lord's feet *intentionally*—including the pains and hurts of previous years—and deliberately focus on God's healing grace in the sacrament, more happens and it happens more often.

Often as a way of focusing on these truths, I picture my burdens inside a large trash bag that, as I kneel down to receive Communion, I leave at the feet of Jesus. Then I picture Jesus extending His hands toward me with a small treasure chest of blessings. While I certainly can have hopes as to what blessings that chest may contain, and can even ask Him for blessings I believe I need, it would be inappropriate for me to try to picture the contents. My Lord knows far better than I do which blessings I need and in what order I should receive them. Only rarely could my determination of what is in the blessing box equal what He has placed there; most of the time my choice would be much inferior to His. In my picturing I leave the box closed and let Him open it and show me what is in it if He chooses to.

Yet sometimes these efforts are not enough. Being conscious of the problem, sharing it with others, prayer and holy Communion always help but perhaps not sufficiently to free us from what is hurting us. It is at this point that many in a prayer and healing ministry give up in frustration or else fall back on the belief that maybe this particular person is not supposed to be healed. I would like to suggest three additional steps. These steps illustrate the fact, by the way, that we must never isolate the ministry of the healing of memories from other aspects of the healing ministry, or indeed from any aspect of the faith.

5. Forgive others.

Often people block their healings—whether physical or emotional—by clinging to resentment. Early in my ministry of healing I ministered to a man who had been sexually abused as a child. I prayed at some length with him over a period of time but saw no change. Finally I gave up. Several months later he called and said he was healed. I asked him how it had happened. He told me that others had ministered to him after I did. One day one of them asked him if he had forgiven the person who had molested him. "No," he responded. "I hate him!" He was reminded that our Lord tells us to forgive others and pray for those who persecute us

(Matthew 5:44). Indeed, Jesus said that if we do not forgive others, we ourselves will not be forgiven (Matthew 6:15). Forgiving the man who molested him had not been easy, but it had brought healing.

Remember, the ministry of the healing of memories should never be an occasion to excuse bad behavior or attitudes. Inner healing recognizes that even though much of a particular problem may be attributable to the sins of others, any part of it that is due to *our* sins has to be confessed and repented of. This includes any sinful responses or attitudes we allow because we were hurt. (The steps to forgiveness are covered in chapter 5.)

As Leanne Payne wisely points out in *Restoring the Christian Soul through Healing Prayer,* "The failure to forgive another is a most formidable barrier to wholeness."

6. Submit to a ministry of deliverance, if needed.

Some emotional problems seem to resist all efforts at healing. In some instances a demonic stranglehold prevents the person from becoming free. Sometimes he or she might have been involved in the occult. This involvement has to be renounced, of course, before progress can be made. Sometimes during the course of a traumatic event, the individual was momentarily susceptible to the demonic, perhaps even calling down spiritual forces on those tormenting him. Sometimes a curse has been placed on the individual. Sometimes Satan chooses to demonically oppress a person who is suffering emotionally. Whatever the reason for or intensity of the demonic activity, deliverance prayer could be necessary at some stage in the inner healing process. (See chapter 7.)

7. Seek professional Christian counseling.

Those whose abuse was major and prolonged may need, in addition to prayer, extensive work in counseling with a capable, wise, caring therapist to understand what happened and how it affected them. Often victims of abuse need a gentle, gradual rebuilding of their lives if deep and lasting change is to occur. These people's whole lives were ordered around a lie and it takes time to reorder each aspect around the truth.

Although God sometimes graces such a person with dramatic progress, it is wrong to demand such progress of a person when God is not giving it. That would have the effect of re-victimizing the victim—shaming him or her for not being whole at a rate that we, and not God, determine.

Christian Imagining

One vehicle that can help us turn over to God the deep-seated hurts of our lives and receive divine healing is Christian imagining—the experiencing of Christian truths in the imagination. (We have already looked at one example of imagining in laying our burdens at the feet of Jesus while receiving holy Communion.) This is not a required step in the healing process, but for some it is very helpful *provided we keep it within Christian boundaries.*

God is a God of beauty and of drama. Jesus often communicated truths not in abstract, philosophical ways, but in story form. His parables were truths easily pictured in the mind's eye—as anyone who has ever acted out a parable knows. Sometimes at a youth group retreat, for example, in order to dramatize how Jesus forgives our sins as we confess to Him, I recorded a few pretend gossipy thoughts on a tape recorder. Then I played the tape to the youngsters to let them see how unconfessed sins are "part of the record." After this, I "confessed" to the Lord that my gossip was wrong, that I would try to make amends and that by His grace I would do better the next time. Then with a tape eraser, representing the cleansing and forgiving power of the Lord, I erased the tape. When we played the tape again, it was blank. The sins were gone! This exercise has proven effective in driving the point home to others—and to myself!

The healing of memories is similarly helped by such imaginings. We might sense Jesus standing with us at the time of a tragedy or feel Him hugging and consoling us. Or we could picture ourselves laying the garbage of what was done to us at His feet for disposal. We can grasp His love for us by picturing Him smiling at us or feeling His arm around us, or just sensing the warmth and security of His presence protecting and freeing us.

We must be cautioned, however, that there is a big difference between this Christian imagining of scriptural truths and the kind of visualization popular in New Age or secular self-help programs. For one thing, proper Christian imagining is always based on *specific biblical truths,* never on the invention of "truth" or the thought that one can bring reality into being by simply picturing it or thinking it.

For another thing, we let God be sovereign in the process. Like many others, I have made use of imagining in ministry by encouraging the hurting individual to picture walking along a beach on a warm, sunny day. Way down the beach a figure appears who is not recognizable immediately. Eventually, however, it becomes apparent it is Jesus. He comes up to the individual and talks. So far, so good. We may have made it easier for a person for whom Jesus has often seemed far-off and remote to talk with the Lord. I might ask the person I am helping in this exercise, "What are you saying to Jesus and what is He saying to you?" If God shows me something at the time or gives me a word, I share it, asking the person what it means to him or her. At this point, however, I step out of the way. For me to go further and tell the person what to say or, worse, for me to make up what I would like Jesus to be saying, is unwise.

God has given us in His Word a rich history of dreams, visions and experiences of being caught up into heaven (like Paul's experience described in 2 Corinthians 12). But historically in Christianity this is something *God* does. We can set the stage with beautiful music, worshipful atmosphere, theological reminders, personal witness or, in this case, by imagining a scene on the beach. To go further is to go beyond how God has led His people through the centuries, to get into the habit of projecting onto God our own thoughts and desires and to play God in the lives of people.

Also, we are careful in this process to make sure that Jesus—the Jesus of Scripture—is the One we seek. A few in the Christian inner healing movement have said it does not matter whom we picture. What counts is the exercise, the imagining itself. Nothing could be further from the truth! While there may be some psychological benefit from an exercise in which someone other than Jesus is imagined, Jesus is the only One who can truly make us whole. He alone has the power, and true wholeness occurs only in relationship to Him. Whatever emotional release may occur in imagining a scene with someone else is paltry compared to the blessings of a deepening relationship with the Lord of the universe. In addition, in picturing or calling out to other spiritual entities, we could be opening ourselves to demonic forces.

And, finally, we make sure to check the veracity of any vision, word or experience against the Scriptures. John reminds us to test the spirits to see if they are from God (1 John 4:1). Thoughts from our subconscious, ideas subtly suggested by others and impressions given by the evil one may all intermingle with genuine communications from God. Hence, we will never take and run with anything that comes to us in such an inner healing exercise without making sure that it squares with what God has given us in His written Word.

At the same time, however, we must be careful of going too far in the other direction. There have been a few best-selling books of late that would have Christians turn away from *any* form of imagining as being New Age. The authors of some of these books belong to a Christian tradition that is highly rationalistic. Nearly everything in their spirituality, in other words, is oriented around the intellectual content of the faith. Their tradition offers little or no awareness, much less intentional practicing, of affective (that is, nonrational) learning, of mystical prayer, rapturous worship and so on.

A closer familiarity with the history of Christian spirituality will teach us the difference between proper, legitimate, time-tested Christian mystical experiences and the New Age, magical, occultic variety.

In his book *Reincarnation,* Mark Albrecht gives a good definition of appropriate mysticism:

> [I]n its classical sense, mysticism may be defined as the seeking of the experience of the presence of God, or union with God and his will. Needless to say, these concepts are quite biblical. So, in that sense we may say that God calls all believers to be mystics. Christianity has a rich heritage of orthodox mysticism and pietism. . . .

We must be careful we do not fall off either end of the table—accepting any imagining without careful discrimination or rejecting it in any form.

There is much from our pasts that continues to affect us negatively today—physically, emotionally and spiritually. As we bring these hurts before the Lord, we can be set free to be the people we want to be and God wants us to be.

A Few Additional Notes of Caution

In the five years since I wrote the first edition of this book, there has been a growing concern that the ministry of inner healing is being misused. We should not be surprised at this. Anything that is good can be twisted. Anything centered in God will be counterfeited when people seek to experience God's blessings in ways detached from Christian discipleship. Anything that combines healing with responsibility will be subject to attempts to substitute blaming others for accepting personal accountability. Let me underscore three things to beware of, three cautions we must hold before us lest the good ministry of inner healing be turned into something that it is not. Please beware of:

Victimization

Even secular commentators note how widespread is the invoking of one's being a victim in order to avoid personal responsibility. If I am not happy, it must be the fault of those who raised me. If I do not get ahead in life, it is because other groups in society have conspired to keep people like me oppressed.

The psychiatrist Erik H. Erikson (1902–1994) argued throughout his life against the prevailing belief—the legacy of Freud's teaching—that the ego is fixed in early childhood. Erikson's belief is that the formation of a person's identity is a lifelong process. "If everything 'goes back' into childhood," he stated, "then everything is somebody else's fault, and trust in one's own power of taking responsibility for oneself may be undermined."

There are several problems, of course, with the cult of the victim. First, it is not always someone else's fault when things do not turn out the way we had hoped. The hard knocks of life deal all people blows. The bad choices we make eventually have their consequences. Unless we are asserting that people are helpless, then we, faced with real obstacles, can choose to respond either by cursing our fate (and blaming others for it) or by seeking ways to overcome these obstacles.

Second, a claim of victimization is often selective and self-serving. That is, some who are quick to claim victim status for themselves are just as quick to deny it to others. More than once I have witnessed an argument between a man and woman in which the woman sought to justify her rude behavior by asserting that all men deserved nothing less for the way men treated her in the past. It did not matter that this particular man had done nothing harmful to her. He was a man, so it was right for him to suffer for the sins of his group. Nor was the woman willing to accept the idea that rude behavior directed toward her by a man was equally acceptable if it was payback for all the harmful things women had done over the years to that particular rude man. Once when

I pointed out these things to a woman, I was told point blank that women can only be victims, never victimizers.

Although this particular example is an issue of sex, such "we-are-victims-you-are-victimizers" attitudes exist in other categories of society. Third, such a claiming of victim status offers no hope. If one's chief self-definition is that of victim, and if one wallows perpetually in the hurt and anger of real or imagined past harm, the focus is backward, not forward. There is no future for such an orientation. The apostle Paul could acknowledge terrible things that happened to him because he stood for Christ; yet he urged both himself and others to forget what lay in the past to press onward to what lay ahead (see Philippians 3:13–14). Not only is Paul's statement God's marching orders to us; it is a statement of good news. Things *can* get better for us if we let go of pity and blame.

We must be careful in the ministry of inner healing that, while not trivializing the real and tragic cases of victimization, marginalization, bigotry and the like, we do not unwittingly encourage the rampant cult of the victim. Rather, we must acknowledge that, yes, terrible things may have happened, but now it is time to forgive, take responsibility for the rest of one's life under the grace and guidance of God and move on.

False memory syndrome

With the explosive growth in the popularity of therapy sessions to "uncover" repressed memories of traumatic events alleged to have happened in childhood, notes of caution have come from many quarters. Although some "uncovered memories" do square with the facts as verified by independent witnesses, there is a growing awareness that some of the "uncovered memories" are not accurate recollections of what happened.

Why is this? One reason has to do with the therapist (or, in our case, the minister of inner healing). Some people, in their inexperience, inability or zeal to help, plant suggestions clumsily or inadvertently in the mind of the client. Such suggestions can work their way into one's subconscious and come out later as "memories." The recent conviction of a day care center worker on charges of child molestation was overturned when the alleged victim later related how certain parts of her testimony about what had happened were suggested to her by a social worker. The alleged victim was not at all sure things had happened the way her parents and social worker had said, but they, as responsible adults, must be telling the truth, so the youngster testified accordingly.

A second reason for caution has to do with the agenda that various people have. Therapists and ministers of inner healing have issues about which they are concerned, even angry. At times, whether subconsciously or deliberately, they can project their views onto their clients, who then "remember" things about their past. It is being reported that a significant number of clients who uncover "memories" of certain kinds of victimization in their youth are the patients of therapists who themselves were victims. In many cases this can be explained by noting that such therapists would have tremendous compassion and affinity for their clients, and such compassion and affinity would make them more sensitive and capable in the process of recollection. It has also been noted, however, that more than a few therapists use their clients to get back at a class in society (men, women, the rich, the powerful, etc.) by suggesting things to their clients that simply did not happen.

Recently the retired Roman Catholic archbishop of Davenport, Iowa, was accused by two women of molesting them thirty years earlier. The plaintiffs' "memory" of the events had been recovered during therapy. But not only was the case dropped for lack of evidence; the therapist herself became a defendant in lawsuits brought by three other women. The charges, denied by the therapist, were medical malpractice, psychiatric negligence and fraud.

A third reason for caution is that we are all bombarded daily with various horror stories of this or that person being subjected to this or that brutalization, victimization or horrid experience. I wonder how much of this information seeps into our subconscious mind, perhaps to be reworked as dreams, symbols or "recollections."

I once ministered to a man—let me call him Charlie—who was convinced he had been rescued as a youngster from a terrible fire. Careful research indicated that no such thing had happened to him. What *had* happened was that while he was reading at home one evening during his childhood, a television account in the background described a most horrible fire and how someone was rescued by a brave firefighter. We—Charlie's family, Charlie himself and I—now theorize that while most of Charlie's attention was on his book, a small portion of it was listening to the background television account, although he himself was not consciously aware he was doing this. Charlie is a sensitive soul and something deep within him was deeply moved. The news account and his inner emotional response were "filed away" in his memory banks. Much later, as an adult, Charlie was troubled by some difficulties at work, making him especially vulnerable to painful thoughts and feelings rising to the surface. Charlie's concern for his work situation somehow coupled with that fire story and produced in Charlie the belief that he had been rescued from a fire.

The point is, be careful about taking as literal any "hidden memory" that you or someone to whom you minister claims. Maybe the event happened, maybe it didn't. While taking the person in ministry seriously, we do not necessarily take literally the details.

This is important. Too many therapists (or ministers of inner healing) have suggested courses of action that *might* (please note, I said *might*) be appropriate *if* the memory were accurate, but would not be appropriate at all if it were not. Earlier in this chapter I cited the example of the woman who was standoffish to her uncle. Somehow her unexplained feelings were that this man had not been nice to her when she was little and that she would be wise to stay away from him lest he do something else harmful. When she discovered that the root of these feelings was his trying to take away a can of toxic chemicals, she learned that her standoffishness had been based on a misunderstanding. If we decide to avoid someone, go public with accusations or call the police because of a newly discovered "memory," how tragic things might be if we are wrong!

The "inner child"

This term has gained considerable popularity, both in Christian inner healing circles and in secular and New Age pop therapies. Once again we must be careful to determine what is meant by those using the term, for there can be considerable differences in meaning. In the sense that "inner child" represents a person in his or her youth, with the various experiences of love and nurture, hurt and abuse, it is a legitimate term. It describes the legacy, good and ill, we all have from our earliest years, including time spent in the womb.

In the sense, however, that there is deep within us an innocent, pure core being, someone who could profitably be listened to for guidance and direction, the term *inner child* contradicts biblical truth. Why is this so?

First, we are to listen to Christ and believe and rely only on the truths of His written Word, Scripture. If Jesus wanted us to listen to our inner child, He would have said so. When Jesus commended the little children and told us to be like them, He was telling us to emulate their trust in Him (Matthew 19:13–15), not to listen to them for guidance and wisdom.

Second, our inner child is not so pure. One need only observe children for a few minutes to see they can be cruel, mean and self-centered. Historically theologians have used the term *original sin* to describe the fact that even from the moment of conception, all of us, except for Jesus Himself, are tainted by inherited sin. To this inherited sin comes actual sin, the sin we commit of our own choice. No person on earth except for Adam and Eve before the Fall, and Jesus in His entire life, is free from such conception-to-grave taint.

Third, if our inner child is so pure, why are we concerned to go back to those moments in our earlier life when serious damage was done to us that affects us today? "In counseling," Leanne Payne rightly reminds us in *Restoring the Christian Soul,* "it is important to realize that the way of the wounded 'inner child' is so often the way of the foolish child. . . ."

The ministry of inner healing is a wonderful ministry when kept within the bounds of biblical revelation. When one transgresses those boundaries, serious and harmful difficulties will occur.

Discussion Questions

1. What is the purpose of "healing of memories"?
2. How is healing of memories different from forgiveness?
3. If you suspect that you may need this type of healing, what should you do?
4. How can you make your imagination available to God?

Experiment

Block out *at least* twenty minutes of quiet solitude. The purpose of this experiment is to make your imagination available to God. Take at least five minutes of quiet, thoughtful, verbal thanksgiving and praise. As you read Isaiah 40, think about the images God gave Isaiah, and what a joy it must have been for Isaiah to receive these pictures in his mind's eye (imagination). Take at least five minutes to imagine yourself as a person described in verse 31. Record your experiment in your healing notebook.

7

Satan, Demons, Temptation and Oppression

The human mind and heart raise basic questions about eternal things. Is there a God? If so, what is He like? What is the purpose of human existence? If there is a purpose, what is God's response when we fail to live up to it? Why is there harm and destruction in the world? If God is good and caring, what will He do about such things?

These basic questions are raised by people of every culture and age. The answers given by the various religions and philosophies differ markedly from each other, a point we should remember the next time someone tells us that "all religions teach the same thing." First we will look at a Christian understanding of evil in the world, then contrast it with what some other religions and philosophies have said.

A Christian Doctrine of Evil in the World

Christianity affirms an eternal God. In His love, before He created the heavens and earth, God created a variety of other beings—angels, principalities, dominions, powers and so forth (Ephesians 6:12). Some, if not all, of these spiritual beings were given free will. While a majority of angels used their free will to remain loyal to God, a minority led by their leader, Lucifer, rebelled (Isaiah 14:12–14; Jude 6). Now called demons, these fallen angels and Lucifer, now called the devil (which means "accuser") or Satan (which means "adversary"), seek to spread the rebellion against God and try to inflict harm against God's people. Jesus said Satan was a murderer from the beginning and the father of lies (John 8:44).

We human beings, also given free will, succumb at times to Satan's various ploys to entice us to join the rebellion, as illustrated in the tragic fall from grace of our protoparents, Adam and Eve (Genesis 3:1–6). Adam and Eve's sin had serious consequences for the world, as we saw in chapter 1.

Yet this is not just Adam and Eve's story. This is the story of us all. We have inherited from Adam alienation and fallenness. To this "original sin" we add our own. As Scripture reminds us, "All have sinned . . ." (Romans 3:23).

All this alienation came about because of our rebellion against God and His ways. Amazingly God, because He is love, nevertheless wishes to rescue us from sin and its various consequences.

He started this mission of rescue first by choosing a people to be especially His. Through the revelation of His will via the Law and the prophets, God taught the Jews what was forbidden and what was expected. He told them (Deuteronomy 18:9–14) to have nothing to do with the various abominations the Canaanites practiced, such as divination, sorcery, mediumship, magic (Genesis 41:8; Daniel 4:7) and astrology (Isaiah 47:13). These were forbidden and against God's will because they involved the guidance and power of spiritual beings not submitted to God, and because they eventually harmed the people who used them.

The best the people of the Old Testament could do in their battle against Satan was attempt to contain the problem by putting to death anyone following the devil's ways (Exodus 22:18; Leviticus 20:27).

Jesus Christ's birth, ministry, atoning death and resurrection demonstrated and effected the beginning of God's final assault against Satan, an assault that will continue until our Lord's return to inaugurate the new heaven and new earth (Isaiah 65:17; 2 Peter 3:13; Revelation 21:1). With the coming of God to earth as a human being, and the subsequent bestowal of the Holy Spirit on all believers, His power was made more readily available to mankind. Souls could be reclaimed. Satan could be pushed back. Ultimate victory could eventually be won.

On the cross Jesus destroyed the chief weapon Satan had—that people would have to suffer the eternal consequences of their sins. In other words, because Jesus took onto Himself the iniquity of us all (Isaiah 53:6), death for believers, while still painful, now leads not to eternal lostness but to eternal life with God. As the *Te Deum Laudamus,* an ancient hymn, puts it, Christ has "opened the kingdom of heaven to all believers." As Paul told the Romans, "The wages of sin is death, but the free gift of God is eternal life in Christ Jesus our Lord" (Romans 6:23). As he told the Corinthians, the sting of death has been removed (1 Corinthians 15:55).

Jesus established God's kingly rule on earth. As this kingly rule expands via the direct work of God and His work through the ministry of the Church, these things happen: Souls are won for God from the domain of Satan; disease (always directly or indirectly a byproduct of humanity's following Satan's enticements to rebel) is cured; deliverance is obtained from the oppression the devil works against us (Acts 10:38); armor is provided to withstand the assaults of the evil one (Ephesians 6:11–17); and offensive weaponry is issued to help us reclaim territory Satan has captured (2 Corinthians 10:4).

Christ began all this on Calvary and continues His work until His glorious return. While His Father has sealed Satan's fate and put some restraints on his activity, Satan is still allowed some measure of freedom. He is still a roaring lion (1 Peter 5:8) and convincing accuser (Revelation 12:10).

Why? Why didn't God completely remove the (albeit limited) influence Satan has over us? The answer is simple, although not easy to take, especially when we or our loved ones are suffering. A primary reason evil still exists in the world is the sinful misuse of the freedom God has given us. As long as we have this freedom, we will, to various degrees, be agents of Satan's work.

Jesus will deal once and for all with evil at His Second Coming (Revelation 21:1–5). But at that time there will no longer be any chance for people to use free will to turn toward (or away from) God. In order for God to give whoever is alive more time to repent and be saved, therefore, Jesus' Second Coming and the final dealing with the existence of evil have been delayed. Peter put it this way: "The Lord is not slow about his promise as some count slowness, but is forbearing toward you, not wishing that any should perish, but that all should reach repentance" (2 Peter 3:9).

Ultimately, then, the problem with Satan and evil will be solved. In the meantime, we know that Christ's death on the cross has made provision for believers to spend eternity with God in heaven, and that Christ's ongoing work today has equipped us with the power necessary to keep Satan at bay when he strikes at us.

Such is the Christian view of the existence—and continued existence—of evil in the world. But what about other views?

Other Religions and Philosophies on the Subject of Evil

Some religions hold that there is no principle or power of evil at all, that everything that happens is not only approved by God but ordained by God. Whatever happens, a convinced Muslim would respond, "Allah wills it."

Thus, while this God may be powerful, is He really good, at least as we understand goodness? In contrast, Christianity states repeatedly the goodness of God (Mark 10:18; Romans

8:28). It is Satan, not God, who inflicts harm. Although God allows Satan some freedom, He has already made provision for our ultimate triumph over evil in Christ. We could not conceive of God's causing a child to be born with a deformity.

Rabbi Harold Kushner, on the other hand, author of *When Bad Things Happen to Good People*, so desires to keep God good that he denies Him much power. To Kushner, God would like to intervene, but His power is limited, so He cannot.

Kushner has little or no doctrine of Satan as the cause of evil, nor does he have faith in Christ who redeemed us at Calvary and who will ultimately triumph and right all wrongs. All Kushner can give us is a God who is ultimately not God at all, for how can God not be all-powerful? That seems a contradiction in terms.

Another possibility is the beliefs of so-called dualistic religions. They posit two ultimate powers equal in strength, one good, the other evil. These powers alternate in their ruling, with neither ever triumphing over the other.

But this gives the devil more than his due. Scripture reminds us that only God is eternal; that Satan is a creature, albeit a rebellious one; that his power, though real, is limited; and that God, for all that He allows, is still ultimately in control. For all Satan's destructiveness now, "God bats last" and will eventually right all injustices. There is an omega point to which history is marching. Things will not continue like this forever.

Some religions, such as Hinduism, see bad events as the resultant punishment for misdeeds done in a previous life. A key belief is that of *karma*—the reward or punishment for our deeds. Thus, it is payment of karmic debt, not the intrusion of Satan, that underlies suffering.

While such a religious philosophy is gaining adherents among some spiritually hungry people in the West, it is not a religion of good news. For one reason, in such a religion one has become his or her own Savior, an impossible task if we consider honestly how hard it is to be perfect. (See how the psalmist recognized this in Psalm 49:7–9.) For another, if someone is suffering to pay off a karmic debt, it would be evil and unloving to help him. It would set him back on his journey. If someone is lying in a ditch, leave him there!

While Jesus came to do many things, chief among them was to be Savior of those who put their trust in Him. In addition, we see Jesus' compassion illustrated in His life and teaching, a compassion that has led us to minister to others at the points of their need. Note that in countries where belief in karma is the dominant view, nearly all the hospitals are built by either Christian missionaries or natives who have been converted or Westernized.

Some people have said, usually in periods of peace and prosperity, that the solution to the problem of evil is found in education. "Ignorance, not evil power, is the problem," this philosophy states. "Once people are educated, all will be well, for humanity is fundamentally good." Recall, however, the shrewd comment of President Theodore Roosevelt: "Take an ignorant man who is stealing from a railroad boxcar and give him education and you may have equipped him to steal the whole railroad."

The heady and naïve optimism prevalent in the first fifteen years of this century that education would solve all our problems was shattered by the agonizing events of World War I. Theologian Karl Barth's grasp of the sinfulness of fallen humanity was not only far truer to Scripture than the liberal theology in vogue prior to World War I; it was far closer to reality. Why is it that this lesson has to be learned again and again?

Others believe that the ennobling effects of culture will so tame whatever is destructive in us that evil will disappear as culture improves. Thus comes the shock when we see how thin a veneer culture really is and how puny a dam to hold back the raging torrents of evil working in us and through us. In the TV miniseries *Holocaust*, Frau Weiss, the doctor's wife, expressed amazement that "such things should be happening in Germany!" Naïvely she did not realize that culture may stop someone from spitting on the sidewalk but it will not stop genocide.

Still others believe that evil does not exist as an objective reality, that it is simply the absence of good. But psychiatrist Carl Gustav Jung noted that "one could hardly call the things that have happened, and still do happen, in the concentration camps of the dictator states an 'accidental lack of perfection'—it would sound like a mockery."

Scott Peck's bestselling book *The People of the Lie* is one in a series of books in which people discover, often to their surprise, that objective evil does exist. This discovery is often in spite of their educational conditioning. Peck notes in another book, *The Road Less Traveled,* that it is not evil that surprises him, but rather that there is so much good.

Why Is the Christian Answer Rejected by Many, Even in the Church?

Why is it, then, in spite of scriptural teaching (believed and practiced for centuries in the Church) and the lack of satisfactory alternative world views, that many people even in the Church have trouble with the Christian answer to the problem of evil?

First is the argument that the biblical view of Satan and the demonic is nothing more than first-century superstition and ignorance. We would hope, whether as an article of faith or from growing experience, that people would see the Scriptures to be not the gropings of people toward theological understanding, but the inspired revelation of truth by God to us. Along the way to that view, we should at least be careful to avoid the all-too-typical polite put-down of calling an earlier era unsophisticated. Today's urbanized world has generally lost the facility to read weather from the color of the sky, the motion of the trees and the feel of the soil. Have we ing Satan, fallen angels shut out of God's Kingdom, is offensive language. It is offensive not because it is inaccurate, but because it judges and excludes. Thus, whether it is a correct description of reality is irrelevant. It is opposed because it makes people uncomfortable. The label *fundamentalism* is a convenient term with which to dismiss such views.

But hasn't our refusal to search for truth become a different kind of fundamentalism, a different kind of simplistic thinking? As the Rev. Paul Zahl put it:

> Here, perhaps, is a flaw in our church's capacity for pastoral care: for our very charity and riding easy over secondary issues can make us impotent to warn people of the practical, personal dangers that gnosticisms like astrology can involve. Our vaunted tolerance can render us susceptible to a damaging nonsense (*The Anglican Digest*, midsummer 1988).

In reaction to those Christians who turn away from Scripture's teaching, other Christians have made deliverance from demons the major part of their ministry to others, sometimes to the point of ignoring other kinds of ministry. How do we respond correctly?

First, we need to remember that Christ supplies us with various kinds of help in combating Satan. Grace helps us overcome temptation. Defensive armor keeps the arrow stings of the enemy from harming us (Ephesians 6:11–17). The ministry of deliverance and exorcism lifts Satan and the demons from or out of a person (Mark 1:23–26, 34; 3:11; 6:7–13; etc.). Offensive weaponry rolls back Satan from others and society (2 Corinthians 10:4).

Second, we need to keep people from using Satan's activity as an excuse for all bad behavior. Flip Wilson's humorous comment "The devil made me do it" is far too easy. While the devil often entices, scarcely does he compel. However much we may be predisposed to listen to Satan because of our bad upbringing, debilitating circumstances or uncontrollable mood swings, we have the ability to resist. Were this not so, everyone would have an ironclad excuse to be horrible.

While some obsessive-compulsive behaviors are produced by satanic possession and cannot be controlled until after one or more sessions of deliverance, such problems are but a small portion of what is wrong with us. And even when behaviors *are* produced by possession, the person is responsible for seeking deliverance.

Third, we need to make sure our ministry is a ministry *to people.* While the demonic elements are bound and removed, we must always deal lovingly with the victims, even as Jesus did in His ministry. The power Jesus gives us is *for people* and *against evil.*

Any loud shouting or histrionic displays did not come from our Lord or His disciples but from the evil spirits, who were then bidden to keep silent (Mark 1:23–26, 34; 5:1–13).

Anyone involved in a ministry of deliverance must ever bear in mind that the purpose of Jesus' work was to set captives free (Luke 4:18), not to harm them emotionally or to judge them. In setting them free, we set them free unto Jesus. There is no way to release them except unto Christ.

While it is true that overzealous people have often done harm in their immature ministrations against evil, I believe far more damage comes from gentle, polite, overly cautious— and ineffectual—church folk who do nothing. As long as we bear in mind that the direct ministry against Satan is but one aspect of Christian ministry, that the power behind our ministry is God's, not ours, and that our ministry is to model that of Jesus, we will seldom do anyone harm.

Fourth, we need to understand the various ways Satan works on people. A consideration of the rare but real phenomenon of actual *possession* by demonic spirits is beyond the scope of this study. (If you are interested, consult the bibliography for good books on this subject.) Much more common are the experiences of Satan's tempting and oppressing God's people. It is to those topics that we will now turn.

Temptation

The most common way Satan seeks to harm us is through temptation to sin. Such temptation marked the beginning of Jesus' public ministry. No doubt Jesus was still basking in the glow of His baptism, the descent of the Holy Spirit upon Him and the reassuring words from heaven (Luke 3:21–22). No doubt Jesus was eagerly anticipating the important ministry lying just ahead. But first there was the matter of the temptations in the wilderness.

Some today assert that they could never be tempted in any serious way. They believe that because of the power God makes available to us, they would never give in to Satan. How foolish! A disciple is not above his teacher (Matthew 10:24). If the Lord was tempted, a Christian will be, too. It is true that we have resources available to us. John reminds us that "he [Christ] who is in you is greater than he [Satan] who is in the world" (1 John 4:4). Yet we need to remember once again that Scripture warns us to be sober and vigilant because Satan still prowls around like a lion seeking someone to devour (1 Peter 5:8). We should not cower in fear but neither should we be cocky. Temptation happens to everyone (see Matthew 26:41) and *that includes us.*

Why temptation?

We know that God is not the author of temptation (James 1:13), but He must permit it because it does exist. Why does God allow temptation? I believe there are three reasons:

One, to preserve our free will. One of God's great gifts to us is our free will, with which we can make choices. To entice us to choose wrongly, Satan comes with temptations to sin. If we could not be persuaded to sin, how free would we be? We would be like robots.

Two, to reveal to us our weaknesses so we can work, with God's help, to grow in Christ. When we are knocked around by various assaults, we see where we are strong and where we are weak. Every one of us has various "besetting sins" (see Hebrews 12:1, KJV), those weak spots where we are most vulnerable. Satan will naturally try to strike us where we are most likely to be tripped up. If we ignore the reality of those Achilles' heels, Satan can blindside us. If we are aware of them, we can be on our guard.

Three, to strengthen us. The successful overcoming of temptation strengthens us. As we are tempted, we get accustomed to the enemy's ways. This prepares us for future temptation. As we are tempted, we become more proficient in receiving God's help during times of great need. This equips us for battle. As we are tempted, we learn more about how to defeat Satan. This leads us to victory. As we are tempted, we see that we do not have to accept giving in to sin as inevitable. This leads to greater holiness.

Being tempted and, all too often, giving in might make us very discouraged, were it not for four facts:

First, while God allows the tempter to work on us, He places limits on what Satan can do. This is similar to the limits God placed on Satan's assault of Job (Job 1:12).

Second, we are told that we will never be tempted beyond our God-assisted ability to escape (1 Corinthians 10:13). The key word, however, is "God-assisted."

Third, God gives us in prayer, in Scripture, in the sacraments and in one another the help we need to triumph when tempted, provided we make use of these means of grace. Once again, these tools are helpful only if we use them.

Fourth, on those occasions when we do give in to temptation, we find the Lord a forgiving Friend as we confess those sins (1 John 1:9).

Satan keeps at it

Having tried his utmost to defeat Jesus by tempting Him in the wilderness, the devil departed, but only for a while. He came back again right after Peter's confession that Jesus was the Christ (Mark 8:29–33), and again in the Garden (Luke 22:42). Note several things:

One, Satan never gives up. He tried again and again to stop Jesus. Never think you will be finished with the devil just because you have resisted him once. He will try again. Be forewarned!

Two, Satan tries different methods. The temptation Satan offered through Peter and the temptation in the Garden were really the same as the temptation in the wilderness—to win the kingdoms of the world by means other than what God the Father appointed—the redemption of sinners by Jesus' atoning death on the cross. Satan was too clever to try the same temptation the same way, so he put it in a different cast. In the wilderness, the temptation came from Satan himself; later it came through Peter with his worldly reasoning; and later still it came from within Jesus' own human nature. Jesus' human nature was not fallen, for He was without sin. But He, being fully human, did experience the desire not to suffer: "Father, if thou art willing, remove this cup from me; nevertheless not my will, but thine, be done" (Luke 22:42). In the rest of humanity, however, human nature is fallen. This fallen human nature is given the term *the flesh* in Scripture.

When we recall the threefold renunciation of "the world, the flesh and the devil" in baptism, we should understand that these words are more than poetic; they are the three chief modes through which temptation comes.

Three, Satan's temptations often follow spiritual highs. Billy Graham has stated that his worst battles with temptation come right after a successful evangelistic crusade. As we just noted, Jesus' temptations came right after His baptism, Peter's confession of faith and His celebration of the Last Supper. I believe that temptations come right after times of intense spiritual experience for two reasons.

One, Satan delights to be the "skunk at the lawn party." God has just done something wonderful for us or through us. Satan wishes to snatch the victory away.

Two, at moments of spiritual triumph we often let our guard down and perhaps even get our pride up. We think that we are already in heaven, or that we have become so spiritually mature as to be invincible.

Victory

Temptation is for real! We are knocked around. Sometimes we even give in and sin. But in the midst of all this we have a loving and powerful Friend in the Lord Jesus Christ. When the things Satan throws at us make us want to scream, we can meditate on the richness of God's grace and boldly proclaim with Paul, "Thanks be to God, who gives us the victory through our Lord Jesus Christ" (1 Corinthians 15:57).

Oppression

In the spiritual warfare between the forces of darkness and the forces of light, Satan not only keeps up his rebellious opposition to God but seeks to drag the rest of creation down with him. In addition to trying to tempt people to sin, he oppresses us in a variety of ways.

Keeping people in darkness

One of these ways is to keep people's minds dull and eyes blind so they will not respond to the Gospel (John 9:39–41; Ephesians 4:18–19; Hebrews 5:11). Once I was preaching an evangelistic sermon in a small village in the Philippines. It became apparent that nothing was registering in my audience. As I had previously experienced some good results from preaching in that country, I started praying silently while preaching, asking God to show me what the problem was. I felt in my spirit that there was a strong presence of evil there actively keeping people from hearing.

I stopped my sermon and went over to several believing Christians, Philippine and American, who understood spiritual warfare, and asked them to take authority in the name of Jesus to bind whatever forces of Satan were loose. Then I resumed preaching. I could sense a change almost immediately. Most people became very receptive. Several remained behind after the service to profess faith in Christ as Lord and Savior.

We later discovered that a group of occultists had put a spell on what we were trying to do in that service. The spell had reality and power but, of course, God's power—*when utilized*—is more powerful. Our taking authority over the magic spell and our prayers for the people in the congregation did not force people to faith. Christian prayer and the exercise of spiritual authority are not and must never be seen as magic. People still have their free wills. But our prayers and binding of evil powers made it possible for them to hear the Gospel and exercise their wills unfettered by the bondage caused by magic spells and evil spirits.

Not all such resistance to the Gospel is caused by the direct operation of evil spirits. Sometimes resistance is due to human pride and the refusal to bend one's will to anyone, especially God. Sometimes the listener cannot figure out what the preacher is trying to say! Other times the listener is hindered from accepting the message because of hypocrisy in the preacher's life. But on many other occasions the problem is demonic oppression.

Blocking worship

This oppression can also occur during worship. Since our "bounden duty" as well as our joy is to worship God in spirit and truth (John 4:23), Satan will seek to make worship dull and uninteresting, or else encourage the enthusiasm to be a kind of frothy, human-generated emotionalism rather than a Holy Spirit-directed fervor. Good worship should do three things: glorify God, edify Christians and evangelize nonbelievers. Dull or out-of-control worship will do none of these. Thus, the enemy has achieved his objectives of thwarting God's purposes, at least for the moment.

One Friday night at the team "prep time" of prayer before

our healing service it was apparent that "our prayers weren't reaching the ceiling." Often these prep times are special moments of drawing close to God and to each other—wonderful preparation for the ministries we would be leading in the service. But not this night. Finally, Mary Shelton, a wise, experienced layperson on the team, stated the problem out loud: "There's an oppressing spirit here." With that, we took authority and bound it in the name of Jesus. Our word of command was something like this: "You spirit of oppression, we bind you in the name of Jesus and command you to leave this place at once. You go to Jesus for your future fate, harming no one on the way." Immediately our time of worship became rich and full.

Now once again, just as with resistance to the Gospel, let it be said that demonic oppression is not the only reason for dull worship. There are times that we rush to church, getting there at the last minute. We are just not ready to be still before God. Other times, like Martha of Bethany, we are distracted by many things. Or we are just plain tired. Sometimes we would rather go through the motions of religious activity than have a true encounter with God. Satanic oppression must not be a catch-all diagnosis to excuse our faults. But on many occasions the problem is demonic oppression.

Believers and accusations

A third occasion of oppression is in the area of accusations. Satan is "the accuser of our brethren" (Revelation 12:10).

The accusations about us start before God. Satan tries to convince God of our unworthiness—not a difficult thing to do since our sins make us unworthy indeed! But our Savior Jesus Christ's twofold ministry of atonement and advocacy is more than adequate for the task.

Through His atonement Christ took the guilt of our sins onto Himself, suffering in our stead (Mark 10:45; 2 Corinthians 5:21; 1 Peter 2:24). When the Father looks at us, He sees Jesus' righteousness covering us like a cloak and pronounces us sinless in Him (Romans 6:23; 1 Corinthians 1:30; 6:11; Ephesians 1:7). And Jesus is our advocate before the Father, so when Satan gives his half-truths ("They are sinners"), Jesus responds with the whole truth, which sets us free ("They are sinners, but redeemed by My blood").

Since Satan cannot convince God of the lostness of those who believe in His Son, he will try to accuse us directly. If he cannot get us to deny our sins, he will try to get us to wallow in them. Just as bad as pride is false humility, which, in reality, is humiliation. Sometimes, of course, the inability to feel forgiven once we have been forgiven is due to other factors, such as hormonal or body chemical imbalance, psychological difficulties and so on. But we must never rule out satanic accusation as a contributing, if not primary, cause. The remedy is to tell Satan to get lost, for once we have confessed our sins and repented, those sins are forgiven in Jesus.

Satan will also try to stir up accusations between or among believers. I never cease to be amazed at how churches can split or Christians can become estranged over the most inconsequential matters. One church I know split over the color of the new carpet in the sanctuary. Such disruption keeps us from our tasks, gives a terrible witness to nonbelievers and is disobedient to the Scriptures (Ephesians 4:1–4). Once again, pointing out Satan's behind-the-scenes influence in these matters does not excuse sinful human behavior. But it should help us see that we are not wrestling against people but against "spiritual hosts of wickedness in the heavenly places" (Ephesians 6:12) and to be on our guard against such satanic tricks. I have heard several wise people say to churches and to Christians estranged from each other, "Let's not gang up against each other. Let's gang up together against the devil while we discuss these issues as brothers and sisters." As Benjamin Franklin said during the war of American independence, "We must all hang together, or assuredly we shall all hang separately."

Sometimes churches seem prone to constant bickering over many generations about the same matters. I know of one church that three times in this century has had a major division over music. Another always seems to fight over property. Many other churches try regularly to fire their clergy. Even though the details change and the people involved are different, there are surprising similarities to each problem the churches have. I believe that just as there are guardian angels protecting each church (see Revelation 2:8, 12, 18, etc.), there are also attending evil spirits that cause disruption in special areas. They work behind the scenes periodically to influence people to act sinfully in particular ways.

Sometimes in these situations the parishioners see the church as just another human organization to be run like any other organization. They do not see the problem first or foremost as one of spiritual warfare. I recall a case, however, in which the pastor of a church with recurring difficulties called me in for help. He knew about spiritual warfare and knew we had to work together to bind the spirits of division and rancor that were harming his church. Now, of course, this was only the first step. It would not take away the need for individuals to repent, ask for forgiveness and forgive others. It would not take away the need for individuals to vow to settle their differences in the love of Jesus. But we seriously doubted that any of these things could ever happen if we did not address the spiritual problem first, and that was, in fact, the key. It is much like a house fire being fueled by a gas leak. You can fight the fire all you want, but until the gas is shut off, putting out the fire is difficult, if not impossible.

The devil's role in illness

A fourth kind of satanic oppression is through illness. Not all, or even the majority of, illness is directly caused by Satan, to be sure. We may, by being sinfully anxious (Philippians 4:6; 1 Peter 5:7), raise our blood pressure or bring on ulcers;

we may be the victims of the malevolent words or deeds of others and develop fears and insecurities; we may have been taught a distorted view of God and fail as a result to enter into a relationship with Him. Our bodies wear out due to the aging process that became part of the human experience at the Fall (Genesis 2:17; 3:19; James 1:15). The devil is lurking in the background here but satanic oppression is not the direct cause in any of these events.

Some illness, however, *is* directly the devil's doing. Jesus said that the woman who was all bent over was bound by Satan (Luke 13:10–17). This is not a poetic or symbolic way of speaking. Nor can we patronize Jesus by saying He spoke this way as an accommodation to or participation in the ignorance of His time. For one thing, Jesus was always quick to correct people who had a wrong or distorted view of things. He loved people but never met them halfway when it came to truth. Plus, there are many places where Scripture distinguishes illness, including epilepsy, from demon possession. Those early Christians, far from being ignorant or gullible, sometimes had an ability to distinguish between various causes of malady in a far more sophisticated manner than we, despite (or because of) all our high-tech achievements.

Several years ago a woman—I'll call her Kellie—was referred to me. She had been suffering from recurrent epileptic seizures for many years. She worked at a hospital and did not lack for medical care. Her doctors threw up their hands in discouragement, however, unable to help her in any significant way. The discernment of the priest who spoke with her initially was that the epilepsy was demonic in origin. This is not to say that all epilepsy comes from an evil spirit, but he believed that in this case it did. I concurred. (For a description of how discernment works, see chapter 10 on the use of spiritual gifts. For a brief treatment of reasons for concluding that a problem might be demonic in nature, see the end of this chapter.)

In the course of one of our public healing services, I prayed and laid my hands on Kellie's head, quietly commanding the evil spirit to depart in Jesus' name. She started to go into an epileptic seizure immediately. The ushers at our service helped her to a chair and attended to her. After the service she said to me, "That was most unusual! My seizures always come at a certain time each month, never at any other time. But this one was not according to schedule. And at the end of the seizure it felt as though something got up and left me! Am I healed?"

Unless I am "110% certain" God is telling me that someone is healed, I do not say yes. Even then I always refer the person to a physician for medical verification. Otherwise there is the potential for much harm. I simply told Kellie that we should praise God for whatever He had just done, ask Him to continue to work and wait to see if the seizures returned. That was October 1982. We are still waiting! Here was a case of an oppressing evil spirit manifesting itself by directly causing an illness. Discernment is needed to know which illnesses are caused by our sin, by disease, by repressed memories of sins done against us, by bad diet, by evil spirits or by any one of a number of causes.

Oppression in general

A fifth occasion of satanic oppression is the "little nastinesses" Satan throws in our paths. Years ago I was part of a team helping out at a large healing service conducted on Tuesday evenings. Until we learned about satanic harassment, we were amazed at the "coincidence" of how minor disasters always seemed to strike us in the hours right before the service. If anyone's child was going to fall down a flight of stairs, if anyone's baby was going to get diarrhea, if anyone's car was to die, if anyone's mother was to call with bad news, if anyone's teenager was going to act horribly or if anyone's tooth filling was to fall out, it was right before the Tuesday evening healing service! I have heard again and again over the years how similar are the experiences of many healing teams.

The answer is to pray protection over yourself and your loved ones regularly, but especially on those days when you join in ministry. When we started doing this before our Tuesday evening healing services, the number of these little nastinesses diminished significantly.

I learned later that praying protection for ourselves *after* the services was important as well. An individual or healing team that has just concluded a time of ministry is especially vulnerable. There are two reasons for this vulnerability.

First, we are spiritually drained. This means that without prayer we will be much more likely to think and act in an all-too-human way. We will do or say things that we regret, we will get into arguments with loved ones and so on. While we might want to act in a godly way, any attempt to do so will draw on our own efforts and not on the power of God within us. We will be "running on empty."

It also means that any additional ministry we attempt will likely fail, for we will not be ministering in the power of the Holy Spirit but in our own strength. We will, furthermore, be vulnerable to Satan's actions on us—without, as it were, the divine shields of protection up.

These last reasons are why I believe Jesus frequently went off for periods of quiet fellowship with His Father after times of ministry (see, for example, Luke 9:18). His human nature was drained, as His statement in reference to the woman with the issue of blood indicates (Luke 8:46). He needed, as it were, to be "tanked up" again. That is to say, His human nature needed to be replenished by the Holy Spirit.

A second reason we are vulnerable after a time of ministry is that we have angered Satan. He has failed in his attempt to deflect us from ministering God's blessings. In his anger he tries to harm us or inflict us with physical, emotional or spiritual distress. He does this to get us to stop ministering in the future ("It's not worth the pain to minister to others," we might conclude), to discredit us and God's work in the eyes of others ("They claim to be God's instruments, but look at them!" others might say) or just to get his little revenge.

I saw a classic example of this when I was ministering healing in a city in the Philippines. Assisting a team of Americans were several devout people from the Episcopal parish and from the missionary hospital, including Dr. Ron Paschia, a Roman Catholic and head of surgery at the hospital. We had concluded the healing service and spent a few moments praising God for the many healings and conversions to Christ that had occurred during the service. We also took a few minutes to ask the Lord to replenish us in the Holy Spirit and to protect us from what the devil might try to do. As we were leaving the church for a time of fellowship and food, a Jeep full of people drove up. They explained that they were late because they had had a flat tire. They wondered if they could be prayed for anyway.

Most of us on the team were so tired from having ministered virtually all day that we begged off further ministry. (By the way, although our hearts may go out to people in need, there are times when saying, "No, I just can't" is the best response to give, as long as you explain that you are so drained you just have nothing to give.)

Dr. Ron felt he was still "undrained" enough to minister. We left him to pray briefly with these latecomers and went off to our supper. About ten minutes later we heard a terrible squeal of tires and saw people running in the direction of the church. There was the doctor sprawled in the road. As people from the hospital lifted him onto a stretcher, he looked up at me and said, "I forgot to ask for protection when I finished."

A few of the people he had prayed for had been wonderfully healed instantly as he prayed for them. After praying for the last of them, Dr. Ron started walking toward the little restaurant to join the rest of the team. In his spiritual euphoria, he forgot his need to pray again for a refilling of the Holy Spirit and protection from the forces of darkness.

Thanks be to God, Dr. Ron's injuries were slight and he was able to join us for the service the next day. But the lesson of the need to pray protection *after* we minister was firmly grafted onto our minds.

Some might say that Dr. Ron's experience was just a coincidence, and maybe it was. Yet the large number of these "coincidences" happening to people who do not pray God's protection before or after they minister leads many to believe they are much more than that.

While we do not pretend to know all the reasons for satanic harassment, we do know it is real, and the protection of God, while not preventing everything bad from happening, makes a big difference when we ask for it.

How Do You Know the Problem Is Satanic in Origin?

Earlier in this chapter I mentioned a priest's discernment that the epilepsy Kellie suffered was demonic in origin. This question needs to be raised: How can we tell the origin of something that might variously be caused by a biochemical disorder, spiritual disobedience, emotional woundedness in childhood, improper diet, evil spirits or any number of other causes? In one sense, we cannot always tell. The root cause or causes of various physical, emotional and spiritual illnesses are on many occasions too complicated or elusive for exact diagnosis. As we have seen, sometimes this does not matter very much. As we apply various remedies, the problem often clears up, even though we may never know which remedy was the one that actually effected the cure.

On other occasions, correctly discovering the root cause or causes is essential. One reason for this is that these causes may be something other than demonic. An automatic snap diagnosis of demonic activity may harm people by keeping them from confronting the real issues underlying their problems. Sometimes the harm comes by giving people excuses for their behavior ("I can't help myself; Satan has a grip on me"). Sometimes the harm comes by deflecting people from the work they need to do in inner healing or in confession. Sometimes the harm is done by forcing something heroic and dramatic (like an exorcism) when the problem is of less severity. As a physician friend pointed out to me, "You don't schedule brain surgery before they've tried aspirin!"

A second reason for discovering the root cause is the hysteria sometimes associated with the ministry of deliverance. Done by well-meaning but spiritually unbalanced "healers," the ministry of deliverance has frequently frightened people into thinking they are thoroughly and utterly possessed of Satan, when that is not the case. (Compare this to the fright in a person who is told, incorrectly and in an offhand manner, that she has cancer.) There is no need for screaming or jumping up and down. Such antics do not frighten Satan. They may, however, leave people emotionally frightened or spiritually wounded.

Sometimes the harm comes from keeping appropriate medical or psychiatric treatment away. There is a similarity between schizophrenia and demonic possession in several ways: potential for lack of contact with reality; hearing voices or seeing things that are not there; profound withdrawal. While on some occasions schizophrenia is the symptom and demonic activity is the root cause, sometimes schizophrenia is non-demonic in origin. To continue to "exorcise" nonexistent demons while keeping counseling and medicine away harms the patient twice: by keeping away appropriate treatment and possibly by scaring the patient.

An interesting study was done among Christian psychiatrists regarding appropriate approaches to the severely mentally disturbed. Questionnaires were mailed to the 260 psychiatrists and psychiatry residents who, at the time of the study, were members of the Christian Medical and Dental Society (CMDS). They were asked to estimate which of three possible interventions (Bible and prayer, insight psychotherapy and psychotropic medications) would be most effective on seven psychological or psychiatric diagnoses. Their general conclusion, while not ruling out the helpfulness of prayer, was that pharmacotherapy—that is, medicines—is the best way of the three to treat schizophrenia and mania; and that Bible study and prayer are more effective than the other two modalities for the diagnoses of alcoholism, sociopathy, suicidal intent and grief reaction. ("Christian Psychiatry: The Impact of Evangelical Belief on Clinical Practice," in *American Journal of Psychiatry* 1991; 148:90–95. The authors are M. Galanter, D. Larson and E. Rubenstone.)

I am happy to receive such wisdom from people who are both mental health experts and practicing, biblical Christians. Too often Christians have arrogantly dismissed everything in the realm of psychiatry or psychotropic medicines because of too frequent encounters with psychiatrists hostile to religion in general and the ministry of deliverance in particular. I have met open-minded, sincere psychiatrists, on the other hand, who are not at all hostile to religion but who have been turned off to the healing ministry because of the harm done by amateurish practitioners.

When I am confronted with a situation in which a diagnosis of demonic activity is possible, I do two things. First, I make sure that the more regular approaches have been tried and found wanting. That is to say, I almost never pinpoint demonic activity initially as the cause without carefully examining the various possibilities. Has the person had a thorough physical examination lately? Does he or she eat a balanced diet? Has he or she made a good, thorough confession recently? Has someone been working with him or her about inner healing issues? Is the person under the care of a psychologist or psychiatrist? What is the person's spiritual life like? Except in extreme cases, I will not begin an in-depth ministry of deliverance until we have covered these bases.

Second, having tried to rule out demonic activity, if possible, I proceed only if there seem to be positive reasons to

do so. What do I look for? In no particular order of importance:

First, I ask about occultic involvement, whether done
innocently or as a deliberate rebellion against God. (See
Appendix 5 for a partial list of occultic practices.)

Second, I ask if there are close relatives who are practicing occultists.

Third, I ask if the person has called upon Satan, or evil
powers, or spiritual powers other than God and the holy
angels, either for assistance, or to minister healing to another
person, or to render harm to another person, or to cause
something to happen.

Fourth, I ask if the person has knowledge of any curses
having been placed on him or her.

Fifth, I ask the person if he believes there are demons and
if so, what are they like, how do they act, what are their
names? Sometimes I will address the demons quietly: "I command any demons who are present to reveal yourselves. In
the name of Jesus, tell me your names." There is no need for
screaming. It does not frighten the demons; it *may* frighten
the person we are trying to help.

While this approach is biblical (Mark 5:9), it is not foolproof. Some demons play tricks or hide and reveal themselves
only after repeated commands. Other times a responding
"voice" may not be demonic, but an indicator of deep psychological disturbance. In general, though, *if done gently,*
this approach can yield helpful information.

Sixth, I look to see if there are unusual spiritual distrac-
tions or "blockings" that may indicate Satan at work. I look
especially for an unusual inability to confess or praise God. I
do not mean by this the boredom or distraction in worship
that happens even to the most devout. I mean the inability
to take on one's lips the name of Jesus or offer aloud statements of praise.

Let me give you an example. Several years ago I was conducting a healing service in the Chapel of St. Andrew's Sem-

inary in Quezon City, the Philippines. During the service I noticed two students leering at me oddly and making a mockery of the event. When they came up for prayer, I felt a strong sense of evil and foreboding. I asked them both to repeat after me, "Jesus is Lord." Neither could utter the phrase. My prayer partner was the Most Rev. Manuel Lumpias, Presiding Bishop of the Philippine Episcopal Church. Together we commanded the evil spirits in Jesus' name to depart, going to Him for their future fate, harming no one on the way. We continued to do this for about ten minutes. Finally both students blurted out, "Jesus is Lord." With that they fell to the floor, physically and spiritually exhausted.

We learned later that in the years prior to seminary, they had both participated in several occultic healing services in their native villages. They had done this not out of intentional rebellion against God, but because loved ones were ill and none of the Christian clergy in their area believed in Jesus' power to heal the sick today. The lack of belief in the healing ministry on the part of their clergy was expressive of theological liberalism that denied basic truths of the Gospel and was centered in a political agenda of overthrowing the regime of Ferdinand Marcos. No wonder these students were both driven to occultists, and no wonder they were ignorant of the dangers!

These six steps I take in ascertaining whether a person's problem is due, in whole or part, to demonic presence have kept me from making snap, often erroneous, judgments. But although they have proven helpful, they are not foolproof. For that reason, as well as the need not to unnecessarily alarm or frighten, we must be especially careful in how we proceed.

I will leave to the more specialized manuals on spiritual warfare a discussion of full-blown exorcism and focus instead on ministering deliverance. What is the difference between the two? Chiefly one of degree. An exorcism may be called for in someone *possessed* by the devil or by a greater number of evil spirits, by particularly tough ones, or both. Deliverance is for someone *oppressed* by evil spirits, particularly a small number. An exorcism needs far more serious prayer preparation before and prayer covering during the time of ministry; deliverance, while not a trivial matter, needs relatively less. An exorcism always needs thorough follow-up spiritually and psychologically; deliverance, while always needing follow-up, usually needs less. While in extreme situations any Christian may be called on to conduct an exorcism, this ministry is usually best left to those specially called, thoroughly trained and carefully prepared for it; a deliverance prayer can be offered by most Christians.

While these distinctions are not to be seen as technical or foolproof, I hope they provide a working definition between the more "entry level" and the advanced kinds of spiritual warfare.

Ministering Deliverance

Following are the steps to a deliverance session.

Preparation

Unless the situation warrants immediate action, deliverance is best scheduled in advance. The reason: It allows proper preparation on the part of those who will be ministering. I recommend whenever possible that deliverance be conducted by two or three people. Their preparation should be bathed in prayer, especially prayer for protection by the blood of Christ and by the holy angels. They should confess any unconfessed sins and remind themselves of the forgiveness that is theirs by faith in Christ. The reason: Sometimes Satan plants thoughts of unworthiness in our minds or speaks to us audibly during the deliverance session about our sin.

His speech, as usual, is full of half-truths. True, we committed those sins. But if we can say, "But I am no longer guilty because my sins have been confessed and washed away by the blood of Jesus," we can successfully parry the accusations of Satan and continue our ministry undistracted. Sometimes preparation for deliverance ministry includes fasting. We may also want to have others in prayer and fasting for us at the appointed hour of ministry.

Preliminary to actual ministry

Unless it is an emergency, we should spend some time talking with the person needing deliverance. We have already talked with him or her enough to conclude that the ministry of deliverance may be warranted. Now we are talking for other reasons.

First, to offer reassurance. Just as many patients appreciate it when their doctor explains an upcoming procedure, a person about to undergo deliverance ministry is most likely frightened. Many have seen the movie *The Exorcist* or heard stories, real or exaggerated, about the wild things that happen during this kind of ministry. Our job is to calm them and assure them that while some frightening things may happen during the time of ministry, we are not interested in histrionics. We might tell them a little bit about what usually happens during a deliverance ministry session.

Second, to elicit their active participation. In most instances, people are not to be passive in ministry, but an active part of the team. It is, after all, *their* life, not ours, and it would be inappropriate for them to become dependent. We can help them take responsibility for their spiritual walk right now by getting them, as much as is possible, to be active in prayer. While in some cases they might not be able to help (if they are seriously possessed or emotionally exhausted or spiritually empty), in many cases we can get them praying. Sooner or later they will have to renounce any occultic involvement and (re)dedicate their life to Jesus, so why not get them on board now?

The time of ministry

Our words are a simple command to Satan and the evil spirits to depart in the name of Jesus. As believers in the Lord

Jesus Christ, we have authority in His name to cast out evil spirits (Matthew 10:1). Once again, we do not have to shout, because neither Satan nor the evil spirits are deaf, nor are they frightened by such nonsense. What does frighten them is the name of Jesus. This holy name is not magic. When the seven sons of Sceva tried to use it apart from the acknowledgment of Jesus as Lord and Savior, an evil spirit drove them out of the house naked and wounded (Acts 19:13–16). The name of Jesus is a reminder to Satan that Jesus defeated Satan's chief weapon, death, on the cross, and that Jesus' blood makes atonement for sin, defeating the eternal lostness people suffer because of sin.

Be careful of magic. Even done with a veneer of Christian language, the use of magic to cast out evil spirits is trying to defeat the devil by using the devil's tools. I have seen harm done by using incantations; by calling down undefined "spiritual powers"; by attempting to overpower Satan with one's own spiritual strength or "soul power"; by the use of a cross or picture of Jesus, not as an adjunct to calling on the Lord's name but as a magic amulet, however Christian-looking. Some black Pentecostal groups, especially those with strong ties to the Caribbean, make use of enemas. Popular in the 1970s, though thankfully less so now, is a custom in some white, blue-collar Pentecostal groups of asking people to retch out the demons into a paper bag. While any of these less-than-Christian approaches may yield some results (some demons may actually leave), others may enter, invited in some cases by the very approaches used to scare the others away.

I often pray quietly, "I command any evil spirits present to depart in the name of Jesus. You will depart, going to Jesus for your future fate, harming no one on the way."

Sometimes there is a noticeable response—sometimes tears; sometimes deep groanings or sighing; sometimes, though not often, flailing of arms or rolling of eyes.

Occasionally evil spirits will speak. Because they are spiritual beings, they may possess information about one of the ministry team or about anything at all that is correct. The beginner in this ministry may get confused by this. "How did this demon know my mother's maiden name?" Sometimes the demon may remind us of a sin we committed. (This is why a good confession beforehand is helpful.) Sometimes the demon will try to play on our sympathies. One addressed me in a sad, childlike voice: "I never wanted to oppress this person in the first place."

The purpose of any of this communication, of course, is to deflect us from our sole purpose: getting the person free in the name of Jesus. That someone would know Mom's maiden name is interesting but irrelevant. "Be gone, in Jesus' name!" That we committed such-and-such a sin is none of the demon's business. We confessed that to Jesus anyway. "Be gone, in Jesus' name!" That some poor little demon may or may not have joined in his fellows' oppressing of a person is not our concern. "Be gone, in Jesus' name!" In no case are we to enter into a discussion with any evil spirits. We ignore what they are saying and keep repeating the command for them to leave, in Jesus' name.

Often, however, there is no outward manifestation of anything.

How do we know when the task is complete and it is time to stop? Once again, while there is no foolproof answer, here are some things I look for:

First, is my discernment telling me the task has been accomplished? This discernment grows with experience.

Second, does the person to whom we have been ministering now sense a release from bondage, a new freedom within, a removal of whatever he or she sensed was wrong?

Third, is the person now able to do things he or she was demonically prevented from doing before (for example, praising the name of Jesus or confessing that He is Lord)?

Sometimes nothing seems to have changed. There are two possible reasons:

First, we were not wise enough or prayed up enough. We

let the enemy fool us. We attempted to do it in our own strength. Don't be discouraged by this. Even Jesus' disciples had to go back to school when they failed at first at deliverance (Matthew 17:19–21). Take stock of what you may have done wrong, ask God for forgiveness and wisdom, do some more reading on the subject and do better next time. In the meantime, find someone more wise and experienced to help the person you failed to help.

Second, we may need to consider whether the diagnosis of demonic oppression or possession was correct.

Aftercare for the person set free

After the time of deliverance ministry is over, it is important that "aftercare" happens. Immediately after any evil spirits have departed, we need to pray with the person a prayer of (re)commitment to Jesus as Lord and Savior and to be filled with the Holy Spirit. It is not enough for the evil to depart. The good now has to enter in. The reason for this is threefold.

First, for protection. Jesus said that when an unclean spirit leaves a place, unless that space is filled, the evil spirit will return and reoccupy the empty place, accompanied this time by several other spirits (Matthew 12:43–45).

Second, for fulfillment of spiritual desires. In many cases, people got involved in occultic/New Age practices because they were spiritually hungry and either did not know the Gospel or, if they did, did not want to pay the price of following Jesus. If we do not point out the dangers of false spiritual choices—dangers that led to the need for deliverance—and if we do not introduce them to the only One who can satisfy their spiritual longings, they might go back to the same occultic/New Age practices, or find different ones.

Third, and most importantly, for wholeness. Only Jesus saves. Even if the person is protected somehow from the return of the evil spirits, and even if the person feels satisfied and fulfilled in life, if he or she does not know Jesus as Lord and Savior, his or her future destiny will be lostness, not eternal life in heaven. What is the point of being set free from "dis-ease," whether physical, emotional or spiritual, only to lose your soul (see Luke 12:20)?

Aftercare includes other aspects of the healing ministry, too. Seldom does deliverance stand alone. Sometimes there needs to be confession for all manner of sins committed during one's bondage. It is fruitless to argue the degree to which a person was or was not responsible for such behavior, given the power Satan had over him or her. Rather, Jesus offers cleansing for sin and power for growth. Why not take advantage of it? Sometimes I encourage a person to pray, "Lord, I don't know what percentage of this was my fault, but whatever amount was, I ask Your forgiveness. I also ask Your cleansing for everything unclean within me and Your power to help me change. In Jesus' name. Amen."

Sometimes a person needs inner healing. Often bad things happened to us while we were in spiritual bondage. We may have been targeted for ridicule by others because we acted in unusual ways. We may have been emotionally hurt by the demons themselves. We may have been emotionally distressed simply because there is much emotional wounding in society. Whatever the reason, I have never seen anyone set free from demonic presence through a ministry of deliverance who did not also need some degree of inner healing.

Aftercare for the ministry team

Remember, the team needs aftercare as well. Spiritual warfare, even of a moderate variety, leaves one drained spiritually and tired physically. Remember to put some time into prayer, asking God to replenish you. After times of ministry, Jesus often went off for times of replenishment. Additionally, pray for protection. God has used you to roll back Satan, even if just a bit. Satan may try to strike back, to punish you and scare you off from future ministry against him. Pray for protection, and there will be far less likelihood of anything bad happening. Positively, spend some time enjoying fellowship with the Lord, whose instrument you just were.

Discussion Questions

1. What does the Fall of Adam and Eve (original sin) mean to you?
2. What does the Fall have to do with brokenness, healing and wholeness?
3. What do you believe the Scriptures mean when referring to the devil, demons and other evil spiritual beings in the world?
4. Satan's favorite weapon is the lie. Discuss Satan's lies in
   a. the temptations of Jesus
   b. our own temptations
   c. "besetting sins" or compulsive and addictive behavior.
5. What is meant by *spiritual warfare?* How important is it in your life?
6. Why is it important to obtain protection before ministering healing? And afterward?

Experiment

Block out *at least* twenty minutes of quiet solitude. The purpose of this experiment is to expose some lies of Satan and to put on some armor. Take at least five minutes in quiet, thoughtful, verbal thanksgiving and praise. Read Ephesians 4:17–24. Assume a comfortable posture. Relax. Ask God to bring to your mind those things that hinder your effectiveness in prayer and healing. Record these in your healing notebook.

8

Christian Healing
and the New Age Movement

One of the current challenges to Christianity in general and to Christian healing in particular is that collection of philosophies and spiritualities given the name "the New Age movement." In many ways there is nothing new about the New Age movement except for the packaging. Many of its beliefs and practices repeat the Baalism against which the Old Testament prophets spoke and the Gnosticism against which such Church Fathers as Irenaeus had to contend.

Although it is beyond the scope of this book to describe in detail the origins and beliefs of the New Age movement, I will list briefly some of its central beliefs in order to illustrate its infiltration into the church's ministry of healing. (See "Recommended Reading" in the back for books treating this subject in detail.)

New Age Beliefs

Monism

This is the belief that all is one. This does not mean a close connectedness, such as the fellowship we enjoy in our personal relationships with God. Rather, *monism* means "a one-ness of *essence*." That is to say, monists believe there is no dif-ference at all between "creator" and the various objects of "creation" except for an illusory, outward appearance. To a monist, the problem of the universe is not one of sin but of separateness. The parts of the One have become separated and the goal is to get everything back together. This is one element behind many forms of witchcraft. Opposites—good and evil, male and female—must be reunited if there is to be a restoration to Oneness.

God as force

Most New Age groups see "god" (or "the divine" or "the numinous" or "the One") as impersonal force, energy or consciousness. (Recall "the force" from the *Star Wars* movie trilogy.) There can be no personal relationship with this power. One learns instead how to gain access to it. Religious leaders do not help people come to know the transcendent-yet-personal God who has a will for their lives. Rather a leader—who may be called magician, witch, adept, wizard, shaman or guru—seeks to instruct people in gaining and using divine power for their own purposes, whatever they may be.

We are God

The old humanistic challenge to Christianity asserted that no matter how noble or worthy we are, we are essentially naked apes, the present end product of an impersonal time-plus-chance evolutionary process. The challenge of the New Age movement is the belief that we are all gods in disguise, emanations from the once-whole One. Werner Erhard, founder of EST, the Mastery Foundation and Forum, put it this way: "You're God in your universe." The Maharishi Mahesh Yogi, founder of Transcendental Meditation, said, "Be still and know that *you* are God." New Age leaders tell us that we can trust our "inner light" as infallible and that we need no authority—not the Bible, the Church or other people—to tell us what to do or believe.

The Christ Spirit vs. Jesus the Christ

While the old theological liberalism saw Jesus as a human being with a particularly well-developed God-consciousness (but not as God made flesh), New Age spirituality sees Jesus as a manifestation of God but not uniquely so. Rather, Jesus of Nazareth was only one of a number of ascended masters who possessed "the Christ Spirit" in a special way. The founders of all the religions of the world and, indeed, many other people possessed this Christ Spirit. Thus, say New Agers, all the religions of the world teach essentially the same thing, and dogmas and doctrinal distinctions are irrelevant. Nearly all cults use the words *God, Jesus, Christ, the Spirit* and so on but with different meanings attached. For that reason Christians must know the Scriptures, the creeds and, as much as possible, the doctrinal controversies in which the post-apostolic Church was embroiled. Otherwise, we may get caught up in a group or by a teaching that sounds good but is subtly, dangerously wrong.

Salvation through knowledge

According to New Age teaching, it is not our sins but the ignorance of our essential goodness and oneness with the entire universe that keeps us from being who and what we are meant to be. In order to grow and develop—and find healing—we need to break through this ignorance. There are, depending on which of the various New Age groups we explore, various ways to do this. Some include meditation techniques that involve emptying oneself, hearing the wisdom of spirit guides speaking through channels, learning to hear and trust the guidance of one's inner voice, accepting the insights of humanistic psychology, participating in consciousness-raising techniques such as sensory deprivation or mind-expanding drugs, or by learning or experiencing such occult practices as astrology, palmistry or séances. The purpose, in any case, is to gain wisdom presently secret or hidden. (The word *occult* literally means "hidden" or "secret.") The reference is to esoteric, deeper truths known only by the specially enlightened elite.

Biblical Christianity, by contrast, is far more democratic. It can be understood by scholars and blue-collar workers, the brilliant and the simple, adults and even children. In combating a form of Gnosticism, Paul taught that the fullness of the Godhead dwelt bodily in Christ, and that in Christ we have come to spiritual fullness (Colossians 2:9–10). In short, we have it all right before us. There is nothing else to get from God except His grace to live more fully into our discipleship. There is no special teaching about doctrine or morality reserved only for the elite, the specially educated, those who have experienced certain special revelations or those who through their pain have come to a different revelation of God. The basics of Christian doctrine and morality are clearly written in Scripture. The problem is not gaining more information or enjoying exhilarating experiences. The problem is surrendering our minds and wills to believe and obey what God has taught.

Reincarnation

This is the belief that souls will keep coming back endlessly until they are enlightened enough to escape into the core of the One. Connected with this is the belief in karma, a Sanskrit word meaning "the result of our deeds." That is, whatever happens to us in this life is determined by our behavior in previous lives. Through "past life regression" we can learn about previous lives so as not to make the same mistakes. Through gaining knowledge of our "true essence" we may escape the cycle of endless incarnations and meld into the One.

Some of the Bible passages that clearly rule out reincarnation are 2 Samuel 12:23; 14:14; Psalm 78:39; Luke 23:39–43; Acts 17:31; 2 Corinthians 5:1, 4–8; 6:2; Galatians 2:16; 3:10–13; Ephesians 2:8–9; Philippians 1:23; Hebrews 9:27; 10:12–14; Revelation 20:11–15.

These, packaged in various ways, are the basic beliefs of the New Age movement.

While we must be careful that we do not label as "New Age" anything that differs from our own opinions or that bears superficial resemblance to New Age teaching, we must be on our guard that these beliefs do not work their way into the practice of Christian healing. The reasons are twofold: First, because one of the ways disciples of Christ honor Him is by believing what He taught, especially in the face of philosophies that contradict. Second, because wrong belief leads to wrong experience. While we seek to obey God because He is God, we soon discover that His commands are good for us and that anything to the contrary is sooner or later harmful. As Jesus said, it is the truth that sets us free (John 8:32).

Areas to Watch

Here are some areas in which we have to be careful that the ministry of Christian healing not be poisoned by New Age beliefs:

An uncritical acceptance of psychology

Psychology is a broad discipline with many branches. Some of these branches are compatible with the teachings of Christ, some are friendly but contain points that disagree, others are hostile and contemptuous. As we welcome the many positive benefits psychology can bring to troubled people, we must be aware of the dangers. We must be aware of the presuppositions of a particular school of psychology or a particular practitioner of psychology.

Is the revealed truth of the Christian faith believed in, or merely tolerated, or even seen as part of a person's problem?

Is the basis for counseling the Christian view of man: created in the image of God but fallen through sin; in need of a Savior, faith in whom leads to forgiveness; whole only when in relationship with God in Christ? Or is man seen as "come of age," able to be made whole apart from a saving relationship with God in Christ?

Is sin seen as a departure from God's will with serious consequences or as another form of neurosis, foisted on people by religion or parents, to be dismissed as a false and harmful idea?

Christians need not cave in before the supposed authority of psychology any more than we should before any other human authority. God has revealed to us in Scripture the true nature of people and what we need to be whole. We hold these tenets not because "it is our religion," but because we believe they are true. Thus, any counselor who has a different set of presuppositions must be seen as (perhaps) sincere but possibly ineffectual or even harmful. This is not because we are jealous of others in the helping professions—we need all the help we can get—but because we know that only what lines up with reality will ultimately help people.

Closely related to this is the area of self-image. Much has been written on this—from scholarly treatises to mass-market paperbacks—and many in the Church assume the best we can do for someone is help him or her overcome a bad self-image. But two points need to be kept before us.

Some of the negatives we feel about ourselves we feel for good reason. Some of the guilt feelings we have are because of *real moral guilt* before God and humanity. *False guilt* (and religion, sad to say, is sometimes to blame for some of this in people) needs to be exposed for the falsehood that it is. True guilt will never go away, however, until it is confessed to God with full purpose of amendment of life, with promise to make whatever restitution is called for and with the willingness to ask the forgiveness of others.

Pumping up a person with a sense of "You're O.K." is like building a house on a shaky foundation. It may make a person feel confident for a while, but it masks over the deeper issues, problems that will once again come crashing to the surface. I have seen guilty people go to therapy session after therapy session in which others are blamed for problems, biblical morality is denied and belief in sin dismissed as foolish. They continue to go to expensive therapy and are no better for it, condemned to a modern equivalent of Lady Macbeth's endless handwashing—always washing but never getting clean. Thank God for Christian counseling (though be warned that a psychologist who is a Christian does not necessarily practice "Christian psychology") in which those insights of psychology compatible with a Christian understanding of mankind, our problems and our hopes can be used to set people truly free.

Our true image emerges only in Christ. It is as we are related to Him that we take on a new nature and have the tarnish of our fallenness removed. More than twenty years ago I heard evangelist Tom Skinner tell more than ten thousand college students how his conversion to Christ changed his self-esteem. Tom, a black man who hated the put-downs of white racists, nevertheless believed inwardly much of what they said. Not long after he came to Christ, Tom read in 1 Peter 2:9 the description of who a person is in Christ. The next day when a bigot taunted him, Tom turned and said, "Don't you know whom you are talking to? I'm a member of the royal priesthood, the holy nation. I'm one of God's own and Jesus dwells within me!" Not only did the bigot turn and flee; so, Tom said, did his own inferiority complex.

A transformation like Tom Skinner's does not usually happen that quickly. Often a person's sense of worthlessness comes from a whole life of emotional deprivation or abuse.

Sharing the good news of God's unconditional love is a necessary first step in a person's healing, but it is seldom enough. Anyone with a rotten self-image needs more than *knowing about* God's love; he needs to *feel* it and feel it over a period of time. This often happens best as he is loved unconditionally by another human being. As such human love is given, he can begin to understand and experience the infinitely more powerful love of God, which alone can bring the root transformation of self-esteem.

Positive prayer as a way to coerce God

Confidence that God can do wonderful things is important to opening us up to receive those blessings. Jesus was stopped in His desire to bless His hometown people because of their unbelief (Matthew 13:58). James tells us that one of the reasons we lack certain things God wants to give us is that we do not ask in faith (James 4:2).

The Church too often wears a false humility before God, assuming that God seldom wishes to bless us. We take Jesus' statement that He came to give us a life of new and special quality (John 10:10) and substitute stoic resignation as our fate. We put aside Jesus' many examples of healing the sick and instead counsel sick people to cope with their pain. Certainly the Church needs a lot of teaching if we are going to exercise positive, believing faith.

A perversion of positive faith has arisen in the so-called positive confession movement. In this brand of teaching, Christians are taught to make a "faith statement" about something they desire, believing that God is then obligated to go along with whatever it is they have prayed for. In another form of this, we are encouraged to visualize ourselves as we want to be—which is almost always successful with a position of influence and power and accompanying material possessions. By visualizing this, confessing it verbally to ourselves and others and banishing as faithless doubt any thought or word to the contrary, our desires will come true. (For an excellent discussion of the positive confession movement, see the chapter "The Prosperity Gospel" in Charles E. Hummel's book *Fire in the Fireplace: Charismatic Renewal in the Nineties.*)

In various forms, this positive imaging is appearing in medical care (when one is encouraged, for instance, to picture light, energy or "good cells" attacking a disease) and in business (from daydreaming about success in an upcoming sales call to focusing power and energy to gain an advantage over someone else).

There are several problems for the Christian in this way of thinking.

First and foremost, where is God in such a scheme? If we have determined what is right for us and then tell God to go do it, we no longer seek God's desire for our lives and instead see Him as a celestial waiter at our beck and call.

While a positive mental attitude is a significant component in the process of healing, and while visualizing oneself may well be an expression of that, we have to remember that *God* is the source of all health, whatever means He may use. I thank God that on many occasions He did not give me what I so earnestly desired. Although His answer was often different from what I wanted, it was always better. We have to be careful, further, that in the process of forming mental pictures of what we want, we are not unwittingly reaching out to spiritual entities not submitted to God.

Second, the desires so often "claimed" in prayers of positive confession are self-indulgent. I have seldom heard such emotional investment in prayers for peace, justice, the poor or one's enemies. Nor have I heard prayers such as Solomon spoke when he turned down the opportunity to pray for his own prosperity and asked instead for wisdom to rule wisely (1 Kings 3:7–12).

Third, this system of thought leaves little room for suffering or walking in the way of the cross. While I agree that the Church is often resigned to illness, not grasping the words or actions of Jesus, still we are told in the Gospels that there will be suffering, ridicule and persecution for bearing His name. We have the examples of Jesus who had nowhere to lay His head (Matthew 8:20) and Paul who was beaten, shipwrecked and jailed (2 Corinthians 11:23–28). Paul reminds us that it is sometimes *amid* famine, peril, persecution, nakedness and the sword that we conquer, not by their removal (Romans 8:35–37).

The "gospel" of the positive confession movement is religion for a sunny day. It is a severe, punishing gospel. In other words, as long as everything is working according to plan we seem to be worthy practitioners of this message. But when things go wrong, when a prayer is not answered, when we are not rolling in material blessings or enjoying perfect health, the implication is that we are not praying correctly, that we somehow allowed doubt to creep in and ruin everything.

To suggest that to someone who is suffering is as insensitive as the comments of Job's friends, who said that if Job was sick and remained sick it had to be his fault (Job 4:7–9; 8:3–7; 11:3–6, 13–20). Sometimes, to be sure, we do not receive God's blessings because we have done something wrong, or because of unbelief or sin (Mark 2:10–11; John 5:14). But as the account of Job shows, this is not always true. Positive confession teaching ill equips us for times of hardship, nor does it kindly dispose us to Christians who are presently suffering. One man told me, "They deserve to suffer because if they had listened to the teachings on positive confession, they'd be on easy street now."

Fourth, the "technique" of gaining what we want through praying "the right way" is an exercise in magic. Magic, or sorcery, is the attempt to get a desired result by reciting certain words or following certain procedures. The words or procedures are paramount, not God. Our ability to use them, not the grace of God, determines the results.

Is a salesperson simply reminding himself that he has a good product and some skill at his craft when he visualizes a sales call going well? Or is he moving into the realm of believing that his imaging will somehow force the reality to come into existence? If it is the latter, then it is magic.

A few in the positive confession movement even say that nonbelievers can get what they want because the laws of positive confession work for anybody who performs them correctly. I wonder if they ever read about the sons of Sceva in Acts 19:13–16 who tried an exorcism "by the Jesus whom Paul preaches," only to have the evil spirits turn on them for such foolishness. Prayer is not the manipulation of God through technique, but a relationship of love.

Fifth, it perverts the meaning of faith. Faith always presupposes an object of that faith. While "the faith" is a body of truths or doctrines, *faith* is always *faith in* someone or something. In positive confession teaching, faith is not faith in God, no matter how much proponents say it is. If God is so unwise or unloving or unable to be trusted with the needs of my life that I have to tell Him exactly what to do, how can I say I have faith in Him? Dr. Charles Farah, a Pentecostal pastor from Tulsa, Oklahoma, rightly calls this attitude presumption. If all hinges on the correct wording of my faith statement with no doubts on my part, then the faith has to be *in me*—in my ability to phrase that confession correctly and without doubt.

Faith, correctly, is the confident trust in God who has proven trustworthy, and who can be trusted with my needs because He is love. While God delights to have us tell Him what our needs are as we perceive them—what loving parent doesn't let a child prattle on with his or her wish list?—we can rest secure in His wise love. We trust Him who has in store for those who love Him things beyond our desires, much less our deserving. This—not some presumptuous foot-stomping or magical manipulation—is the ultimate faith statement.

Sixth, by denying the reality of lingering symptoms, we have stepped over the line into Christian Science. Christian Science is not just another denomination that happens to stress healing. It is a religious philosophy that denies the reality of material things. In Christian Science, one's body cannot be sick because the body is illusory. The problem is in *thinking* oneself to be sick. Healing in Christian Science is bringing a person to a place of more rightly understanding the nonreality of the problem. Thus, someone who says, "I'm healed, but the symptoms don't know it yet" might be a victim of this dangerous teaching.

Too many operations have been called off, too much medicine has been thrown away, too many people have been harmed by the belief that if we just say the right words everything is healed immediately, no matter what the symptoms indicate. A person is not healed until the symptoms are healed! It is much better to say, "I believe Jesus is healing me right now. I don't know how quickly or slowly He will be doing this, so until the symptoms clear up, I will continue to pray and take my medicine."

Healing through magic

In the laudable growth of the restoration of healing in the Church, we have to be careful that we do not slip into a form of healing that is occult. We have to be on our guard in three areas especially.

First, we in the Church have to be on our guard in terms of diagnosis. We find two methods of diagnosis in Scripture—observation/testing/conversation and a word of knowledge.

As for the former, Jesus or the apostles often saw what the problem was or else the sick person or a loved one told them. Expanding this into current medical practice, we have the intake interview and the evidence yielded by various diagnostic tools such as taking one's temperature or blood pressure, taking an X ray or CT scan and so on. In a session of healing or counseling, the person seeking prayer will tell us what he or she believes the problem to be. The person ministering healing or doing counseling will ask questions to garner further information. Problems in a person's life will often point directly to certain root causes.

The word of knowledge, as we will see in chapter 10, is one of the gifts of the Holy Spirit referred to in 1 Corinthians 12:8. It means a supernatural bestowal of information by God directly to a person. Someone in a healing ministry will often pray with an individual and get a strong impression that something is wrong instead of, or in addition to, what the sick person spoke of. In some cases the sick person knows about the problem and is surprised when the one praying says, "Can we pray for your gall bladder [or whatever] problem, too?" In other cases the sick person does not know he has a problem in that area. Many times the people being prayed for are amazed and thankful when their physicians not only confirm a problem in that area but express gladness that it was discovered when it was.

Those are the two scriptural forms of diagnosis—observation/testing/conversation and a word of knowledge from God.

In occult healing, other means of diagnosis are employed, such as spirit guides speaking through "channels," séances or psychometry (holding an object owned by a person to receive impressions or thoughts). Olga Worrell, a well-known occult healer in Baltimore, receives words from her dead husband now in "the spirit world." Others try to discern illness by becoming sensitive to energy waves emanating from a body.

What is wrong with these practices?

They are occultic, and all occultic practices are condemned in Scripture (Leviticus 19:31; 20:6, 27; Deuteronomy 18:9–14). Followers of Jesus do not wish to participate in anything God rules out, even if we do not always understand why He rules it out.

Also, the power source behind them is satanic. While some occultic practices may look harmless, Christians know that their power source is the devil. Paul tells us that what people sacrifice to idols they are sacrificing, however unknowingly, to demons (1 Corinthians 10:20). We know that Satan can masquerade as an angel of light (2 Corinthians 11:14) until someone has been involved with forbidden practices long enough to get hooked, harmed or both. I have spoken to dozens of clergy of many denominations representing a variety of viewpoints who have told me of the problems that eventually befell parishioners who got involved in occult-based healing services. This has been my experience, too. Problems such as deep, lasting depression, onset of compulsivity in particular sins, indifference to God in those once keen for Him and, in a few cases, a series of bizarre accidents have been observed in those who have made use of healers not following God's ways. Lengthy sessions of deliverance or exorcism have often been necessary.

Second, we in the Church have to be on our guard regarding the means of cure. Christian healing is based on prayers for healing to God who cures. While the whole tenor of Scripture indicates that God is on the side of health—indeed we do not find Jesus ever refusing anyone who comes to Him for healing—God retains sovereignty over what happens. God may heal with no appeal made to Him by anyone. God may heal directly in response to prayer. God may choose to make use of material objects by which grace, blessing and healing are conveyed. In Scripture and Church tradition we read of blessed prayer cloths (Acts 19:11–12) and holy oil (James 5:14). God may use Communion, holy water or any number of objects. The historical term in the Church for these things is *sacramentals.* One contemporary Pentecostal minister of healing has called them "delivery systems." In addition, the laying on of hands is frequently a part of healing—indeed, of many different acts of blessing.

The most crucial thing to remember when ministering to the sick is that the Lord likes to heal in a variety of ways. On one occasion Jesus put His fingers in someone's ears; another time He placed mud on someone's eyes; on other occasions He issued a command to walk, rebuked a fever and simply stated that someone back home was no longer ill.

The reason for this variation in manner of healing is so that *the focus will be kept on God.* Christian healing does not believe God to be capricious. We can confidently offer prayer, administer the various sacramentals and lay hands on the sick. But since we are never certain as to which way God will choose to heal or the time frame in which He will accomplish it, our focus is kept on Him. There is no "technique of healing."

In various New Age healings, cure is effected by invoking spiritual powers or readjusting the flow of energy either from outside or from within. Whether this involves energy emanating from therapeutic touch, cooking up a potion of herbs, rubbing crystals over an infected area or invoking spiritual entities by chanting, the central focus is off the God of Scripture and onto a procedure or ritual.

One might ask why, if our Lord likes to heal in a variety of ways, are these New Age ways ruled out? Is this not an example of ecclesiastical narrow-mindedness? The answer is no.

While God uses a variety of ways to heal, the number is not limitless. God does use a number of ways, but He has ruled out many others. Anyone wishing to perform a Christian ministry of healing will make use of the diversity God allows, while turning from those things He does not. Also, we can corrupt even the means God does use to heal if we focus on them for the healing and not on Him.

Healings can be done through New Age practice. Caring for and tending to another person has salutary effects. The placebo effect can be at work. And one can get in touch, whether deliberately or unwittingly, with demonic powers that initially may bless (though eventually will harm).

But such New Age techniques of healing miss the point. More than our receiving a healing, God wants us *whole.* Healing, whether physical or emotional, is only part of it—and not the most important part. What God wants for us and what we so desperately need, whether we recognize it or not, is a vital and growing relationship between Him and ourselves. Like the rich young ruler, we may be graced with wonderful things but miss the Kingdom of God. If it is wrong to eschew God's more material blessings by maintaining that "He's all I need," it is much worse to have the blessings of earth but not those of heaven. What is the point of going to hell healthy (Matthew 5:29–30)? We certainly can have both—both the Healer and the healing—as long as we remind ourselves regularly of the correct order of priority: "Seek ye *first* the kingdom of God, and his righteousness; and [then] all these things shall be added unto you" (Matthew 6:33, KJV, italics added).

Third, we in the Church have to be on our guard against occult healing in terms of morality. By focusing on techniques, we ignore the strong moral component to Christian healing. If someone is suffering the physical complications of a life filled with anxiety, repressed anger or bitterness, and those attempting to help do not deal with the underlying causes of the illness, they are not helping the individual be more whole as a person. They may just be removing one symptom only to see another pop up at a later date in a different part of the body. While, as we have said, not all physical or emotional sickness is based on one's own sin, some of it is. And all spiritual sickness, to a greater or lesser degree, involves sin.

In light of all of this, what should be said about medical science? Because God is a God of order, our discoveries hold true on a regular basis, even though our Newtonian-Cartesian belief in immutable "laws of nature" is being revised. Because God told us to subdue creation (Genesis 1:28), we have a mandate for scientific exploration, however watchful we must be against polluting and despoiling. Medical science is legitimate. But it, too, must be careful lest it sees a medical cure as all-important, the diagnosis of symptoms (and not root causes) as sufficient and science as God.

Uncritical acceptance that anything unusual is a gift of the Holy Spirit

So many in the Church are starving for direct contact with God or for a miraculous manifestation of God that when something out of the ordinary comes, they sometimes accept it uncritically.

Occultic clairvoyance may be confused with a word of knowledge, clairaudience with the "still, small voice" of God, words of "spirit guides" channeled through mediums as words of prophecy. Yet, while not being duped by such spiritual counterfeits (a false path at best, dangerous at worst), neither do we want to go to the opposite extreme and say that the gifts of the Holy Spirit were only for the purpose of getting the Church going, and that any purported gift of God via special knowledge is satanic.

How can we make use of the gifts of the Holy Spirit while not falling victim to Satan's masquerade?

• By placing ourselves under the protection of God and His holy angels (Psalm 91:1, 11; Hebrews 1:14).

• By asking God to remove any supernatural ability to know, sense, hear or speak that is not of Him and to take firm control of any gift that is innate or of Him.

• By testing any word spoken to us directly or given to us by another against Scripture, the written Word of God. Since God is not a God of confusion (1 Corinthians 14:33), anything said by God now will not contradict the revelation He has already given us in Scripture. Be especially careful to note what is being said about the nature of God; the virgin birth; the divinity, sinless life and bodily resurrection of Jesus Christ; the uniqueness of Jesus; the forgiveness of sin only by faith in Jesus' atoning work on the cross; and the moral/ethical commandments of Scripture. As John said, "Test the spirits" (1 John 4:1). Does the purported message square with Scripture and does it lead to holiness, obedience, love, service?

- By examining the lifestyles of those who purport to speak for God. We do have heavenly treasure in earthen vessels (2 Corinthians 4:7) and will always experience a gap, therefore, between what we are and what we ought to be; but those who speak for God should be a representation of His message in their lives. While we do not want to push this point too far (I remember giving a sermon on gentleness that changed several lives on the same day I got into a terrible argument with a colleague), the life of the purported vehicle of communication must still ring true.

- By consulting the wisdom of the faithful over the centuries. As we read through the history of the Church, we are reminded that we are not the first generation of believers to confront this issue. Throughout the centuries Christians have had to discern the difference between the authentic movement of the Spirit, merely human experiences and various spiritual counterfeits of the enemy. Many such Christians have written about their efforts in discernment. Their writings are extremely helpful to guide us as we similarly have to discern. We ignore such sacred tradition at our peril.[1]

Why This Problem of New Age Infiltration?

A cook can serve tainted meat or poisonous mushrooms and do great harm, no matter how sincerely the food was prepared or how tasty it was to the palate. Careful inspection of our food is wise and necessary. Similarly, New Age teaching can be served up with the best of intent and still wreak havoc in the Body of Christ. But why? Why should some in the Church be so vulnerable to such aberrant teaching?

Spiritual hunger

I have met many people who have gotten involved in dubious or even dangerous groups because their own churches have left them spiritually starving. I have met many who have gone to occultic healing services because their churches neglect or even refuse to have services of Christian healing.

We should not be surprised when a dog raids the garbage pail if we have neglected to put food in its dish.

Itching ears

Scripture tells us (2 Timothy 4:3) there will be times when people will find the regular, solid teaching of the faith boring after a while and run after whatever is new and exciting.

Laziness

Many Christians fail to do the hard work of Scripture study, opting instead for grabbing a few verses out of context or reading magazine articles. Lacking a grounding in the truths of the faith, such people can be seduced easily by something that sounds spiritual even though it is not compatible with what God has revealed.

More to be desired is the example of the Jews of Beroea who, upon hearing Paul proclaim the Gospel, "[examined] the scriptures daily to see if these things were so" (Acts 17:11).

Misapplied tolerance

Jesus, who exhibited and commanded tolerance and love of people, insisted at the same time that error be refuted and the truth be communicated (Mark 12:24; John 8:32). He showed that error enslaves and truth liberates. We understand that in all other areas of life. We do not want dentists to drill our gums but our teeth—and the ones with cavities. We want banks to have our accounts correct to the penny. But when it comes to the truths that Jesus taught, we confuse loving people with believing that their opinions, however contradictory of God's revelation, are just as good as any other opinions. We confuse acceptance of people with acceptance of opinion. As a result the very people we are trying to love are given tainted meat and not led toward wholesome spiritual food.

Self-indulgence

New Age spirituality is morally easy. With the loving and moral personal God of the Bible reduced to impersonal force, and with cure of sickness seen as the redirection of energy rather than being related in some way to lifestyle, New Age teaching offers spirituality without accountability, religion without repentance, blessings without discipleship. A student who learns various ways to acquire secret wisdom, manipulate energy or even cast spells learns to be in charge. For those used to being the captain of their ship and the master of their soul, being in control is far more palatable than submitting to God. A few well-known books purporting to give insights channeled from sages of old are apparently built, though disguised slightly, around torrid love affairs with married lovers. Ramtha, a 35,000-year-old warrior "channeled" by J. Z. Knight, is said to teach no right or wrong, just individual reality.

Power

Church history is replete with examples from medieval popes to present-day TV preachers who use religion as a way to gain power. To a Christian tired of being run-down while a secular neighbor prospers, to a salesperson pressured to produce or to a grievously ill person desperate for healing, the possibility of making reality happen through visualization, positive confession or channeling energy is an alluring temptation.

Satan

As always, Satan offers wisdom (of a sort) and power to those who will fall in with him. Masquerading as an angel of light, he seduces those who might resist him if he looked blatantly evil, and is high-tech enough for those who would laugh off a little man with a pitchfork and stretchy red suit. His desire, nevertheless, is to turn people away from God, whether through outright rejection or through interest in lesser things.

As the movements of renewal struggle to restore sound scriptural theology and recover neglected ministries such as healing, may God grant us both the ability to be gentle and the desire to be firm. May He help us hold fast to what is good and make it more widely available, and show us how to root New Age errors out of the Church.

Discussion Questions

1. Review each of the five New Age beliefs described, and reflect whether you have heard it, in some form, in the context of your Christian community.
2. How would you go about selecting or recommending a psychotherapist?
3. Consider the usual prayers in your prayer fellowships (church, prayer group, etc.). Can you detect the development of techniques, formulas or protocols? If so, analyze them in the light of this chapter.
4. Define "occult practices."
5. What do you understand to be the dangers of occult practices?
6. Can spiritual healing originate outside the Church? Why or why not?

9

The Sacraments as Vehicles of Healing

Christianity is, as we saw in chapter 1, incarnational. That is to say, Christianity is based on the truth that God, who is Spirit, became flesh in Jesus of Nazareth. Christians should have no trouble understanding, therefore, that God can use physical objects as vehicles for conveying various blessings, including healing. The sacraments are some of those vehicles.

Although in the early centuries of the Church a variety of rites and ceremonies were considered sacraments, the number was fixed in the eleventh century at seven. Certain Christian groups today observe all seven. Other Christian groups count only baptism and holy Communion as sacraments. Still other Christian groups observe these two but call them *ordinances*. A few Christian groups do not observe even baptism and Communion. For the purpose of this study, I will look at the seven historic sacraments.

Throughout the centuries there have been unbalanced views of the sacraments as the Church went to one extreme or the other in her understanding of them. I would like to examine three ways in which the Church has fallen, or can fall today, into imbalance.

The **first** imbalance is in treating the physical elements of a sacrament either as magic objects or as mere symbols. In the former case, the physical elements of a sacrament—water in baptism, bread and wine in Communion, oil in unction, etc.—are seen as possessing such power that personal faith in God is unnecessary. In the Middle Ages, for example, some people would bury a consecrated host from Communion in their fields to ensure a good harvest and ward off natural disaster. Personal faith in God was not as important to them as the presence of the sacramental bread, which was seen as possessing magical properties.

On the other hand, and in reaction to this, some see the sacraments as mere symbols, simply visual aids to belief. Many Protestants today would say that this was a much-needed theological correction by the leaders of the Reformation. But this understanding of the Reformation is historically incorrect. While some in the Reformation viewed sacraments as symbols, they were very much in the minority. Rather, it was the Enlightenment era 150 years later that championed this view. The Enlightenment denied *any* belief in the supernatural, reducing Christianity as it did to merely ethical moralism. While most evangelical Protestant churches today have turned their backs on most of the teachings of the Enlightenment and embrace the virgin birth of Christ, the incarnation, His bodily resurrection and so on, they have not similarly restored the dominant Reformation view of the sacraments.

Even in calling the sacraments symbols, moreover, people forget there are two kinds of symbols: *mere symbols* and *participatory symbols*. A *mere symbol* is one that stands for something else, nothing more. A flag, for example, is a mere symbol because it stands for a country. In no way is it that country. A *participatory symbol* both stands for something and, to various degrees, *is* the thing it symbolizes. A dollar bill stands for one dollar's worth of the credit of the United States, but it can also be spent for a dollar's worth of goods. If we are to use the word *symbol* to describe a sacrament, it is this kind of symbol we should mean. A sacrament points to something beyond itself, yet also participates in it in a way that a mental tool cannot.

A **second** imbalance is between the objective and subjective parts of a sacrament—that is to say, between the objective reality of what a sacrament is and does, and our subjective, or personal, appropriation of God's grace through our faith.

If too much emphasis is placed on the objective reality of the sacrament, it may replace God as the object of our faith. If too much emphasis is placed on the necessity of our faith, on the other hand, we make our weak grasp of God more important than His strong grasp of us. Then, when our faith is weak, we will deny ourselves blessings in the sacraments when we need them most.

After Jesus rose from the dead, two of His disciples met Him on the road to Emmaus, although they did not recognize Him (Luke 24:13–35). They later described how their hearts burned within them during that journey. Although part of this inward glow was because they were discussing the Word of God, part of it was because the Lord was with them though they did not know it. This demonstrates the objective reality of what happens when Christ is present, even when we have no knowledge of His presence. In a similar way, the sacraments are a real blessing, even when knowledge or faith is not present.

The **third** imbalance has to do with how we know God. Scripture tells us to love God with our minds (Mark 12:30). Besides promoting a relationship between a believer and God, Christianity also involves assent to doctrinal revelation. Without this, faith quickly degenerates into subjective experiences and sentimental feelings.

Knowing God through our minds is important, but that is not the only way to know or experience God. People can encounter God in more mystical ways by observing a sunset, in worship, in an encounter with a holy person, even in being "caught up to the third heaven" like the apostle Paul (2 Corinthians 12:1–4), and so on. People can even encounter God deep within their spirits while they are asleep or in a coma. This is not to say, of course, that *any* religious experience is an encounter with God. John tells us to test the spirits to see if they are from God, and God's test is a doctrinal one (1 John 4:1). It is to say, however, that God comes to us in ways besides pondering the truths of doctrine in our minds. One of these ways is through the sacraments.

United Methodist leader Dr. Ross Whetstone has pointed out that Protestantism is the religious expression of the print culture. Protestantism arose and was shaped by the rise of literacy, the explosion of books and the availability of the Scriptures made possible by the invention of movable type in the century preceding the Reformation. As a result, Protestantism has put so great an emphasis on knowing God through the mind that it has sometimes neglected or even denied knowing God in other ways. When we consider the superstition rampant in Christianity in late medieval Europe, we can understand this. It is, however, an imbalance.

What is needed, as always, is balance. Scriptural revelation always judges personal experience, but personal experience helps us understand scriptural revelation in ways that go beyond (but never contradict) what we know in our minds. Or, put another way, God heals as the forms and elements of the sacraments serve as object lessons of scriptural truth and lead us to personal faith, but God also uses the sacraments to heal and bless when our minds are tired, weak or distracted.

Three Objections to the Sacraments

As with anything else in the Christian faith, objections are raised to belief in the sacraments. Let me list and respond to some of these objections.

Objection #1: The sacraments are just "dead religion."

We have all witnessed the administration of a sacrament that was spiritually lifeless. But is that the fault of the sacraments, I would ask, or the fault of those leading and participating in the service? Non-sacramental worship can be "dead religion," too. So can a Bible study. The important thing is for those involved to see what the sacraments can be. Later in this chapter I will quote extensively from a wonderful book *And Their Eyes Were Opened: Encountering Jesus in the Sacraments* by Michael Scanlan and Ann Therese Shields. The authors, a Roman Catholic priest/university president and a nun, give a wealth of practical help to those wishing the sacraments to be what they are supposed to be, life-changing encounters with Jesus.

As for the sacraments being "dead," remember that God is in the resurrection business, not the funeral business. If something is wrong, God wants to change it. If it is dead, God wants to make it alive again.

Objection #2: Traditionalism is an enemy of the Gospel and the sacraments are traditional.

There are two answers to this objection. First, the Lord Jesus was not opposed to traditions. He told His followers to repeat the Lord's Prayer. He instituted the Lord's Supper to be observed until His return. Our Lord's objection to tradition was when it was used to deny God's truth (Mark 7:11–13).

Second, there is a difference between *tradition* and *traditionalism*. Lutheran historian Jaroslav Pelikan has pointed out that tradition is the living faith of the dead, while traditionalism is the dead faith of the living. That is, tradition is the goodly and godly heritage passed on from previous generations to those alive today, while traditionalism is people today going through religious forms either with no faith or as an attempt to keep faith at a distance. Traditionalism is clinging to forms so that God will not come close. Yes, the outward expression of the sacraments can change. From time to time churches revise their forms of worship. Different forms of worship can express various aspects of the truth inherent in a sacrament. Different ways of worship minister to people with different preferences in worship style or with different personality types.[1]

It is helpful to see a sacrament as wine and the forms as the wineskin. As the power of God in the sacrament comes to us as new wine, the wineskins—the outward forms—may often need to be changed. It would be incorrect, however, to denigrate the sacraments as being old wineskins worthy only of being thrown out. Many churches of all types are realizing the truth that the sacraments are important and central to the faith. Many churches, which until recently had observed Communion infrequently and as a mere symbol, are now observing it more often and as something far greater than a mere visual aid to faith.

Objection #3: The sacraments look Catholic.

I hope God's people will see this for the unbiblical prejudice that it is. Christians of all persuasions are learning from each other. Just as many Roman Catholics are learning to study the Bible as evangelical Protestants do and are expressing the spiritual gifts as Pentecostals do, non-Catholic Christians can rejoice in a fuller participation in the sacraments.

Let's now take a look at the sacraments and see how they relate to Christian healing.

Baptism

As for baptism, Scanlan and Shields say this:

> In Baptism, an adult, or a child through his parents, by the power of the Spirit, rejects the kingdom of darkness as hav-

ing any authority to rule his life. He accepts the kingdom of light and is consecrated and dedicated to the Lord. The sacrament empowers the individual to live and move in the victory of Jesus Christ, won for him on the cross. The community welcomes the person and pledges responsibility to incorporate him lovingly and supportively into the body of Jesus Christ.

The Jews learned the need for formal incorporation into the community of faith when God instructed them to circumcise their sons on the eighth day after birth. The early Christian Church saw baptism as the new covenant fulfillment of the old covenant rite of circumcision. Although most of the baptisms described in the New Testament are of adults—they were the first generation to hear and respond to the Gospel, just as Abraham was the first Jew—there is ample evidence for acknowledging baptism as something also right and proper for the children of believing parents.

Honest differences exist as to the appropriate time for the rite. Nevertheless, infant baptism is much more than a little ceremony to celebrate the addition of a baby to the family. It is the time when the Church incorporates a child into the covenant community of faith. When the Philippian jailer put his faith in Christ, not only he but his whole household was baptized (Acts 16:33). Similarly, when Lydia, a seller of purple goods, came to faith in Christ, "she was baptized, with her household" (Acts 16:15). We have copies of services for baptism from the late second century in which, after the adult converts were baptized, children and infants had their turn. Far from arguing for this practice as if it were some innovation or perversion of the original order, that liturgy simply states that this is what is to be done. From this, most scholars have inferred that baptism was administered to the children and infants of believers from the earliest days of the Church.

In any case, to be thus brought into covenant relationship with God is the greatest healing possible. While anyone baptized as an infant has to go on to embrace Christ as Lord and Savior in a mature, adult commitment, infant or believer baptism signals the removal of an individual from the kingdom of darkness into the Kingdom of light.

Let me illustrate with the story of some friends of mine, Father Philip Zampino and his wife, Jean. Their young son, Mark, was having a tough time sleeping at night. It seemed that something was terrorizing him. They had been waiting for a convenient time to have Mark baptized, but after prayer the Lord revealed to them that they should not postpone Mark's baptism. They went ahead in obedience, and immediately after Mark was baptized, he began sleeping through the night. This was one of many experiences the Lord used to show the Zampinos that, as Christian believers, they had not only the privilege of bringing their children into the covenant of faith and, therefore, out of the world of darkness, but the duty to do so.

Most liturgies of baptism include a prayer of renunciation of Satan and his forces. Some churches include a prayer of exorcism that any evil powers oppressing or possessing the person being baptized will be driven away by Christ. This was especially important in the early centuries of the Church when many had been involved in occult practices before they came to Christ. With the rise of the New Age movement and Satanism in our day, these prayers in the baptismal service once again take on urgency.

Holy Communion

The service of holy Communion is also called the Eucharist, divine Liturgy, the Mass or the Lord's Supper. After Jesus rose from the dead two of His disciples encountered Him on one occasion as He broke bread with them. In Luke 24:30–31 we read how their eyes were opened as He did this and they recognized Him. This was the Lord's way of reminding them that although He was soon to ascend back to heaven, they would continue to encounter Him as they repeated the Lord's Supper. In Acts 2:42 we read that one of the marks of the ongoing life of the Church was the breaking of bread, another way of describing a service of holy Communion. Along with lessons based on the teachings of the apostles, fellowship and prayer, Communion was to be a regular occurrence in the life of the Church. This is why, from her earliest days, the Church observed Communion as a regular part of Sunday worship and not just once yearly, on the anniversary of Maundy Thursday.

Commenting on holy Communion, Scanlan and Shields say this:

> In the Eucharist, we can expect to be healed each time we receive—healed physically, spiritually, and empowered to deal with those relationships and situations of that day with Jesus' wisdom and love and strength. We are given those gifts in his body and blood. . . . Finally, through the Eucharist, we are drawn into deeper personal union with him who is Lord of our lives.

The apostolic and post-apostolic Church recognized Communion as a means of healing. In fact, for them Communion, not anointing with oil, was the chief sacrament of healing. When anyone was ill, deacons would bring the consecrated elements to the sick person's home directly from the Sunday Eucharistic celebration. They would continue this until he or she recovered. People were encouraged to see that receiving Communion was not only good for them spiritually; it was also a way to be blessed and healed physically. Father Ted Dobson in *Say But the Word* (Paulist, 1984) writes,

> . . . In the earliest Christian days, the Eucharist was seen as a sacrament of healing and transformation, a rite that brought wholeness to the people who celebrated it. For example, St. Augustine in his greatest book, *The City of God,* as well as in

his last book, *Revisions,* witnessed to the healing he had seen in his own church as a result of people receiving Eucharist.

When the elements are consecrated—that is to say, made holy, or set apart as vehicles through which God sacramentally blesses, feeds and heals His people—we are reminded that Jesus Christ offered Himself on Calvary to forgive our sins and open up other blessings to believers. The historic words of the Anglican liturgy bring home this point forcefully: ". . . Through faith in His blood we . . . have remission of our sins *and all other benefits of His passion*" (italics added). One of these benefits, of course, is healing. Barbara Shlemon Ryan noted in a leaflet "The Healing Power of the Eucharist":

> Each time we attend the [Eucharistic] celebration . . . we are at a healing service. As we approach the altar, we pray, "Lord, I am not worthy to receive You, but only say the word and I shall be healed." This is a prayer of confidence in the power of Jesus Christ to transform our physical, emotional and spiritual needs. If we truly believe that Jesus is present in the consecrated bread, then we should expect to obtain wholeness as we accept His body into ourselves.

Over the years I have seen many people healed as they receive Communion. Lest we think this is simply because they are using Communion as a time to plead with God for their needs, let me hasten to add that in some cases people were not asking God for anything. Several people told me later they were thinking of what they were going to do after church was over! God had used Communion sovereignly as a vehicle for healing people who needed it, even when they were not paying particular attention.

It is important, therefore, to see the objective nature of holy Communion. In many Protestant circles until recently, Communion, though deemed important, was celebrated infrequently. Simple reminders of Jesus' work on the cross, after all, can be given in lots of ways besides the Lord's Supper. But when one starts to discover—or, better, rediscover—the lost truth that receiving Communion is, in and of itself, important and beneficial, one will desire such feeding far more regularly. In Roman Catholic circles until the liturgical renewal that accompanied Vatican II, Roman Catholics went to mass weekly (or more often) but seldom received Communion. The focus, as with Protestants, was on *hearing* the events of Calvary, but not *receiving* those benefits sacramentally. Now it is much less likely for a Roman Catholic to go to mass and not receive Communion.

In the closing prayer, blessing and dismissal of a Communion service, we ask God to equip us to go into the world to be His blessing to others. This reminds us that while our relationship with God must be personal, it is never private. We are to bring His Word, His love and His healing to this broken and hurting world.[2]

Confirmation

If in infant baptism others made promises to God on our behalf, in confirmation we take these promises on for ourselves. Having asked Jesus Christ to be our Lord and Savior, we ask the Holy Spirit to empower us to be obedient, effective disciples of the Lord. As Scanlan and Shields put it:

> In Confirmation, we accept responsibility to live in the body of Christ and to support it by those gifts God has given us. The church confirms that those gifts are truly of the Spirit and empowers and calls us to use them for service. We are now witnesses of God's love and power in our lives. We can testify to it through our ministries, and the community of the church pledges to support our growth.

There is a connection, as we have seen, between sin and sickness, obedience and wholeness. As the Holy Spirit strengthens us to obey, we find our lives more whole and, frequently, less sick. With the tremendous needs all around us, God wants his disciples to go forth to minister in a variety of ways, including healing. Confirmation is a time for this strengthening and equipping. We read in Acts 19:1–7 how the laying on of hands by Paul was the occasion for the Holy Spirit to fall on a group of people who then spoke in tongues and prophesied.

While confirmation for many people is little more than a fancy joining of a church, when it is done right, it is that special time of empowering that God intends it to be. Let me share the story of one such service of confirmation I was privileged to witness.

During the middle 1970s one of my tasks as a staff member of St. Timothy's Episcopal Church, Catonsville, Maryland, was to prepare adults for confirmation. One year I had an exceptional class of approximately sixty people. During the classes I stressed not only the various events of Church history and the various customs and particularities of our denomination, but especially the centrality of dedicating one's life to Christ as Lord and Savior and receiving the empowerment of the Holy Spirit for discipleship and service. Just about everyone in the class was looking forward to the service as an opportunity for public witness to their commitment to Christ and as a time to be strengthened by the Holy Spirit.

The bishop who was to do the confirming was the Rt. Rev. William Cox, a most godly man who himself knows the Lord and the power of the Holy Spirit. (In fact, Bishop Cox has a nationally respected ministry in leading healing missions.)

As it turned out, that service was a powerful witness to the reality of the Holy Spirit. Nearly everyone confirmed was "slain in the Spirit" (see Appendix 1). Several spoke in tongues for the first time, a few received visions, others prophesied. A number were healed physically or emotionally. It became apparent afterward that many had been given various gifts of the Holy Spirit for ministry, including gifts of healing.

A number of people who had been to confirmations many times before commented on how unusual the service was that evening. My response was that while the service may have been different, we should not have seen it as abnormal. In other words, although we may not have seen this kind of service before, what we witnessed that evening was the norm, the way confirmation is supposed to be. When individuals are making a conscious commitment to Christ and seeking the Spirit's power, and when the one presiding knows first-hand the importance of these realities, results will follow.

Notice the tie-ins to healing. First, profession of faith in Christ as Lord and Savior brings the greatest healing of all—reconciliation with God. Second, other kinds of healing may take place. Third, some receive one or more of the healing gifts of the Holy Spirit. Fourth, others receive different gifts that, while not specifically healing gifts, assist the ministry of healing (see the next chapter as to how this happens).

Roman Catholic scholars Kilian McDonnell, OSB, and George Montague, SM, have published an exhaustive study of the writings of Christian authors in the first several centuries after the apostolic era.[3] The evidence is overwhelming that baptism in the Holy Spirit was integral to Christian initiation. The conclusion drawn for today is that if we are to be faithful to the beliefs and practices of the primitive Church, we must view baptism in the Spirit not as belonging to the private piety of those so inclined, but as normative in the life of the Church and necessary for each Christian.

Penance

This sacrament was, until recently, popularly called *confession* but is now usually called *reconciliation*.

We have already seen in chapter 5 the connection between confession of sin and healing. Confessing our sins, as with anything else, can be either a mechanical ritual—to satisfy an obligation or make us feel good—or else a life-giving reality to help move us toward holy living and selfless love of others.

Father Michael Scanlan told me once that in the early years of his priesthood, hearing confession had become, as for many priests, a duty to endure. Many coming to confession rattled off a list of relatively trivial sins while avoiding more serious root attitudes. Occasionally, however, someone would present himself or herself for confession with the desire to do serious business with God. Father Mike noticed that in many cases, such people were healed physically, either right there in the confessional or else shortly after making their confessions. These experiences helped him to see both the reality of the ministry of healing and the riches offered in the sacrament of reconciliation when done seriously.

As the word *reconciliation* implies, the focus is not solely unburdening oneself from guilt, but also reestablishing the fellowship with God and others that has been broken through sin.

Another step toward healing is the assurance of pardon as we confess our sins, for God is indeed faithful and just and cleanses us (see 1 John 1:9). As our consciences are cleared from guilt, we know that, in spite of our imperfections, God wishes to use us in service to others. As Scanlan and Shields put it,

> In Penance, we now know that to be holy is first to desire and experience forgiveness. The sacrament is a life-giving experience, not an act of condescension on the part of God. In God's healing presence, with the gifts given the confessor and penitent, we can discern the root of a sin, know that it can be destroyed and know that the pain can be healed by his power.

Holy Matrimony

Because so many weddings we attend are really secular weddings held in a church building for social reasons, we may lose sight of what matrimony is intended to be. In a Christian marriage God binds two people together in Him in a special covenant. The Protestant reformer John Calvin, who rejected much of late medieval Roman Catholic sacramental theology, numbered matrimony as a sacrament along with baptism and Communion.

As two people become one in Christ, God pours out His grace, that their love may heal any emotional wounds brought to the marriage. Hurts and insecurities are ministered to and each person becomes more whole. As this happens, they become a sign to the world of the transforming and healing power of Christ.

I give glory to God that He has given me in my wife, Mary, not only a special companion and fellow minister, but a person who ministers healing to my own various emotional hurts.

As Scanlan and Shields state,

> In Matrimony, God anoints two people to be the sign, the tangible witness of the way he loves and is united to his Church. Two people make public their desire to lay down their lives for one another in love, to so be for the other that their love can encourage and support and be a sign of hope to the whole body. Their covenant, made public by the sacrament, is to become a reflection of God's covenant of love with his people. The sacrament so empowers them to give their lives to one another that they are made one. That physical and spiritual union is a concrete sign of God's desire to be one with his people.

Unction or Anointing with Oil

James 5:14 states: "Is any among you sick? Let him call for the elders of the church, and let them [anoint] him with oil." We don't, of course, want to limit God to working healing only in this way. I recall a woman once asking me to anoint her for healing. When I told her that I must have left my anointing oil at home, she replied, "Never mind. I'll be ministered to another time." Although I tried to assure her that God could heal without the oil and that we could pray for healing nevertheless, she said she would rather wait until I had my oil with me. She had confused *one* way of healing with the *only* way of healing.

On the other hand, while God can use a whole variety of means to heal, we should never rule any of them out. On another occasion a man told me, "You can pray for my healing, but don't anoint me with oil. I'm not into that sort of thing." My response to the man was that while there is nothing magical about the oil, the statement in James 5 *is a command:* If you're sick, call for the elders to anoint you. If he was not willing to submit to that, he was placing a roadblock in God's way, and perhaps that refusal was blocking his healing. He responded that he never thought of it in that way before, and he consented to my anointing him. He was healed immediately! Why God's way to heal him had to be through anointing, I'm not certain. I do suspect, however, that it was God's way of teaching him that in order to seek God's blessings, one cannot tell God how to go about His work.

In this sacrament we have the opportunity to receive God's blessings for healing. Listen to the expectancy in Scanlan and Shields' description of coming to this sacrament:

> In the Anointing of the Sick, we can experience in our need the most loving thing God desires to do for us. We *expect* that to happen to us and to those for whom we gather to pray as they receive the sacrament. We expect to see the sick restored to health . . . we expect to see those [so] called [to] approach death with joy and total confidence.

Recall how at the beginning of this chapter we discussed both objective and subjective elements of a sacrament. Sometimes we depend too much on the personal faith of those ministering and need to remember the other side—the objective nature of a sacrament. A good example of God at work in the sacraments apart from individual worthiness came in the Church in the fourth century during a time of persecution of the Church in northern Africa. Some Church leaders caved in under persecution. Many in the Church wondered if the sacraments performed by these weak leaders were valid. If their leaders were that weak, after all, how could God use them? As the Church sought the mind of the Lord on this, God showed them that the unworthiness of the minister does not hinder the efficacy of the sacrament. This belief has been part of the Church's faith ever since, and rightly so. No one is worthy enough to minister the sacraments, teach the Scriptures or lead the flock. If spiritual blessings depend on the worthiness of the leaders, no one in the Church could receive much of anything. God wishes us to know that His promises in the sacraments are not dependent on the foibles of men but on His faithfulness.

Let me illustrate this in regard to anointing. Often at a healing mission I tell the people present that while I will be happy to anoint them for healing, I would like them to ask the clergy of their home churches to anoint them as well. When people respond that their clergy have never done this or even make fun of the idea of anointing, I respond that they should *insist* on it. Some have called or written to tell me that they received a healing not when I prayed for them, but when the leaders of their own church prayed! In more than a few cases, the clergy did this primarily to get their parishioners off their backs and were as surprised as anyone when it actually worked! God honored the sacrament regardless of the faith of those ministering it. In some cases this was the occasion for those ministers to come to believe in the power of God to heal.

Ordination

This is the setting apart and empowering of individuals that God has raised up for ministry. Scripture uses the terms *bishops, elders* and *deacons*. This includes clergy known today as *ministers, pastors* and *priests*. We see in Scripture that from the earliest days of the Church, individuals were specially empowered with spiritual gifts (1 Corinthians 12, Ephesians 4, Romans 12), and individuals were raised up to the office of bishop, elder and deacon (1 Timothy 3, Titus 1). It is not a case of spiritual gifts *or* ordained clergy, but both spiritual gifts *and* ordained clergy. Both are scriptural. As Scanlan and Shields say regarding ordination:

> In Holy Orders, a person is called into a special order within the body of Christ. It is a uniquely holy position, for he is called by the community which has supported his gifts and life . . . to call forth adoration and praise. As that person has grown, the members of the Christian community recognize that they can place special confidence and trust in him, [and are] hereafter responsible for what [they have] nurtured, called forth, and confirmed. He who accepts that call is empowered by the sacrament to lay down his life for God's own.

The sacrament of ordination relates to healing in at least four ways:

One, as we have already seen, clergy are ministers of healing by virtue of office. James 5:14 does not say to call for those elders who also possess a spiritual gift of healing, but simply to *call for the elders*. By virtue of their office, they have a sacramental ministry of healing.

Two, the ordained leadership of a Christian community possesses a disciplinary role. The purpose of church discipline is always restoration of an offending individual to the community and to godly living (Matthew 18:15–20). While we are not to obey spiritual leaders who ask us to believe something that contradicts the clear teaching of Scripture, on all other occasions God calls us to submit to His authorities. On several occasions my submission to authority has led me to renounce certain sins I might not otherwise have renounced. To repeat, there is a connection between sin and sickness.

Three, the ordained leadership has a pastoral role to the flock. As the leaders bring us comfort and counsel, we come into greater wholeness.

Four, Ephesians 4:11–12 includes in the definition of the role of the pastor/teacher the equipping of the saints for the work of ministry. It is their task to help identify those being raised up by God to minister healing, to train them and deploy and supervise them for this ministry. (This is spelled out more fully in chapters 11–13.)

Yes, the sacraments have often been ministered wrongly or experienced as ineffectual. But that can be said about everything else in the life of the Church. Our task is to ask God to restore lively sacramental life in the Church and to work toward that restoration. God's provision for our wholeness through the sacraments is great, and so is our need. As Scanlan and Shields remind us, the sacraments promise "the gift of grace we seek, healing, nourishing, cleansing, freeing, consecrating, blessing, empowering us to accept His reign in our lives and deepen our covenant with Him and His people."

Discussion Questions

1. How does the Enlightenment complement Christianity?

2. How does the Enlightenment undermine Christianity?

3. Think of an example of God touching you or someone else by means of (a) intellect, (b) emotions, (c) imagination, (d) memories and (e) will.

4. Which of the above are purely rational? Which are non-rational?

5. If God speaks to us through all five of these aspects of our being, in how many ways have you been neglecting to look for Him?

6. For each of the sacraments discussed in this chapter, answer two questions:

a. What symbolism is involved?

b. In what ways can the symbol legitimately be the thing it symbolizes?

Experiment

In anticipation of a celebration of the Eucharist, read about the early Passovers in the Old Testament (see Exodus 12:1–28; Leviticus 23:4–8; 2 Chronicles 35:10–19; Ezra 6:16–22.) Ask God to enable you to participate with Old Testament believers in a Passover. Anticipating another Eucharist, read about the Last Supper (Luke 22:7–30). Ask God to enable you to participate in that meal. Anticipating still another, read about the Marriage Feast of the Lamb (Revelation 19:1–9). Ask God to enable you to participate even now in that meal. Reflect on the Passover and the Marriage Feast of the Lamb during the liturgy, while partaking of Communion and afterwards.

10

Ministering Healing
Using the Spiritual Gifts

In order to help us minister healing effectively, God has given the Church various spiritual gifts. These gifts are mentioned in several places in the New Testament, usually with an encouragement to use them: "Having gifts that differ according to the grace given to us, let us use them" (Romans 12:6); "To each is given the manifestation of the Spirit for the common good" (1 Corinthians 12:7); "'When he ascended on high he led a host of captives, and he gave gifts to men' . . . for the equipment of the saints, for the work of ministry, for building up the body of Christ" (Ephesians 4:8, 12); "As each has received a gift, employ it for one another, as good stewards of God's varied grace . . ." (1 Peter 4:10).

What is a spiritual gift? Dr. C. Peter Wagner of Fuller Theological Seminary, author of the bestselling book *Your Spiritual Gifts Can Help Your Church Grow*, starts each definition of a gift with these words: "The gift of _____ is that special ability that God gives to certain members of the Body of Christ to. . . ." We certainly need God's help if we are to render effective service to others and glorify His holy name.

It is often pointed out that between the two chapters on the gifts of the Spirit in 1 Corinthians (chapters 12 and 14) is a chapter on love. From this, some conclude that the Corinthian Christians needed to be reminded to exercise the gifts of the Spirit *in love,* lest they become a "noisy gong or a clanging cymbal" (1 Corinthians 13:1). That conclusion, I believe, is not only correct but as much needed today as it was then. We have all seen people with great ministry ability hurt the people they were trying to help by ministering in an insensitive, unloving manner. We have also seen people use spiritual gifts to gain improper control over others. Anyone who wants to use the spiritual gifts must use them in love.

Yet the reverse is also true. The chapter on love is given in the context of spiritual gifts. Love is much more than sentimental feelings, noble intentions or words of pity. Love includes rendering help to a person in need. To say that we love someone when we do not provide practical assistance is hollow and possibly also hypocritical. So while the love chapter tells us how to use the gifts, the gifts chapters tell us how to love. I find it no coincidence that in each of the major lists of spiritual gifts in Scripture (Romans 12, 1 Corinthians 12–14, Ephesians 4 and 1 Peter 4), there is also a statement about love. To give God's love, we must use God's gifts.

How Do We Receive the Gifts?

If the spiritual gifts are important for effective, practical, loving ministry, how do we come by them? I believe there are two ways:

First, we can offer the abilities and talents we have had all our lives to God for Him to correct and use.

When I was five years old I climbed onto the piano bench and played the first several notes of the song my grandmother had just played. My parents and grandparents concluded that

I had musical talent, so piano and, later, organ lessons were arranged. At age sixteen I started assisting on the organ in a church with a venerable men and boy's choir. I believe I did adequately. At age twenty, my commitment to Jesus Christ deepened significantly. I consciously laid my music at the feet of the Lord, that He might correct anything that was wrong and use my ability as He saw fit to His honor and glory. After church the next Sunday, several people remarked how differently I had played that day. They could not explain what they meant. I had not played more accurately, nor were the stop registrations different. But all seemed to agree with the statement one person made—that I played "more worshipfully." By asking God to be in control of my music, I believe He was more able to use it for His purposes.

I have heard similar stories from artists and sports figures.

We have many abilities or talents that have been with us all our lives. We call them natural abilities, although, of course, they come from God. As we offer them to God for correction and control, we find that He will use them more directly for His purposes.

The **second** way we acquire spiritual gifts is by a direct, sudden intervention of God, either in response to a request or as a sovereign act.

Let me illustrate this with the experience of a friend of mine. Bertha (let's call her) is a fine woman and a deeply committed Christian. She lacks the ability, however, to read people or situations. As her husband put it, "Bertha is a fine lady with zero street smarts." Then one day while praying with someone, she had a profound insight into that person's problems. She knew it had to have come from God. Far from being an isolated incident, this ability continued. Soon people at her church were marveling at how well Bertha could detect root problems in people's lives. God had given her a spiritual gift—in this case, the gift called the word of knowledge.

As long as our motives are to serve others and glorify God, it is not wrong to ask for spiritual gifts. In fact, when a Christian realizes the call of God to minister in His name, he or she should ask God for the tools to do that job better. Whether rededicating ourselves to Christ or committing to good stewardship, whether alone or in a group, a request for additional spiritual gifts is always in order. We might ask God in this way: "Dear God, I know You want me to serve Your people effectively. I know that I can bear no fruit in ministry without Your grace. I ask You to give me those gifts that You want me to have, so I may fulfill that ministry to which You call me. Please keep me from using these gifts to my own glory or in a manner that harms others. In Jesus' name. Amen."

Objections to the Gifts

Not everyone thinks we should get involved with spiritual gifts. In fact, some people warn that this is a risky business. Given the encouragement in the New Testament to use the gifts and the evidence that they can help people and glorify God, why do they oppose their use? I have found three reasons:

The **first** objection comes from the fact that the spiritual gifts are misused. They see someone getting proud and self-important because he or she is being specially used by God. Or they see someone using spiritual gifts in a way that harms others. It is a terrible misuse of the gift of prophecy or the gift of knowledge to go up to someone and bowl them over with, "God has given me a word for you. If you are wise, you'll listen to what I have to say."

In addition, they see the gifts used in such a way that other blessings of God are ignored. They see someone paying more attention to a word God has given him than he does to Scripture. They see someone refuse medical treatment because she demands a miraculous and instantaneous healing.

The proper response to this objection is to say that just because some people treat the gifts incorrectly is no reason to stop using them. Anything good can be misused.

A **second** objection to the spiritual gifts is the belief that they were only an interim measure, to be used for only a brief period in the life of the Church to get it established. We looked at this objection briefly in chapter 3. Let's now consider it more fully.

Scripture does not seem to place a time limit on the use of the spiritual gifts. We read in Mark 16:17–18, "And these signs will accompany those who believe: in my name they will cast out demons; they will speak in new tongues; . . . they will lay their hands on the sick, and they will recover." Nothing suggests that this promise is only for a period of time.

First Corinthians 13 states that prophecies will pass away and tongues will cease (verse 8), but verse 10 explains that the imperfect will pass away "when the perfect comes." It is obvious that this cannot refer to the establishment of the Church, for the Church is far from perfect. Nor can it mean the final writing of Scripture for, although Scripture is perfect, we know from Church history that the use of the spiritual gifts continued as a major part of the Church for a long time afterward. Nor can it refer to any other event, for things are not perfect now. Many commentators see the phrase *when the perfect comes* to mean "when the *perfect one* comes"—the Lord's Second Coming. So, yes, the gifts will cease, but not until they have no further purpose, when Jesus returns.

The purpose of the gifts is to bring God's intervening love to particular situations, not just to expand the Church. While it often happens that people who are miraculously healed then become disciples of Jesus, the Lord's motive in healing, according to the Gospel writers, is primarily compassionate love, not evangelism (see Matthew 14:14, for example). The prophetic word given by Agabus that there would be a famine (Acts 11:28) gave Christians time to plan a course of action to respond. The usefulness of this divine warning had nothing to do with how well the Church was established. The writer of Hebrews reminds us (13:8) that Jesus Christ is the same yesterday and today and forever. We should not be surprised, therefore, that His love for us continues to be expressed through the spiritual gifts.

While it might make a convenient theory to say that the gifts of the Spirit died out after the Church got going and are, therefore, not available to us today, the fact is they did not die out! It is true that they *died down,* but that was because the Church became a religious establishment, not because the gifts had no further purpose. As we read Church history, we discover that whenever faith flourishes, such supernatural occurrences again become widespread.

A **third** objection to the spiritual gifts is really more an objection to the theology and culture that have grown up around them than to the gifts themselves. That is to say, many are put off by the "packaging" in which they see the gifts expressed. This is the same problem some people have with the sacraments.

For the better part of this century, most of those who champion the cause of the spiritual gifts have stressed that a Christian must have a distinct post-conversion experience of grace called the baptism of the Holy Spirit. Many believe that the evidence of this having taken place is the ability to speak in tongues, and they point to several places in the book of Acts where tongues evidenced the reception of the Holy Spirit and/or conversion to Christ.

Without getting into the whole issue of this particular theological viewpoint, let me point out that I have known many people who have been used greatly in spiritual gifts who would claim neither a distinct experience called the baptism in the Holy Spirit nor the ability ever to have spoken in tongues. Certainly Billy Graham has the gift of evangelism. He ministers unquestionably in the power of the Holy Spirit. Yet Dr. Graham has stated several times that he has never spoken in tongues. Many Scripture scholars would say that what we see before us in Acts is a *description* of what happened to some people, not a *prescription* of what should happen to everyone else.

In any event, it boils down to this: We should not reject the use of the spiritual gifts just because we do not necessarily accept a Pentecostal understanding of the baptism of the Holy Spirit. Christians with a variety of understandings of this subject are today making use of the spiritual gifts, with good results.

As for culture, many who stress spiritual gifts also express their Christian faith in a particular cultural style. Sadly, many who do not like that style turn off to the spiritual gifts as well. In other words, if the only context in which someone sees the spiritual gifts being used is a loud, demonstrative worship service with contemporary music, guitars and synthesizer, dislike of that music and those instruments might put that person off to the spiritual gifts as well.

May I stress that the *cultural expression* of charismatic renewal is incidental to the reality of the spiritual gifts? I have seen the spiritual gifts used in a variety of worship settings, from Pentecostal tent meeting, to formal Presbyterian worship, to Roman Catholic high mass! What is necessary for the gifts to be manifested is an openness to the Holy Spirit's working, not a particular style of worship.

C. Peter Wagner, church growth expert from Fuller Seminary, has popularized the phrase *third wave*. He identifies the first wave of the power of the Holy Spirit, which surfaced at the outset of the twentieth century, as Pentecostalism with its distinct theology and cultural expression; and the second wave as the charismatic renewal, again with its own theology and culture. The third wave that many believe is taking place today is already formulating its own theology and style. In this third wave, Wagner notes, God is enabling churches of many kinds, unaffiliated with Pentecostalism or the charismatic renewal, to incorporate the reality of the power and gifts of the Spirit into what they already know and cherish in their churches. In short, we can honor what God has already been giving to the churches as we receive a fresh outpouring of the Spirit. As a Southern Baptist pastor told me, "I can have the riches of Pentecost without turning Pentecostal."

How Do We Know We Have a Particular Gift?

One way is obvious. Something significant happens as we minister. That is to say, we teach and people learn; we sense that we know some piece of information that we have not studied or been told, and, behold, we are correct. Or we try to straighten out an organizational mess, and things start flowing smoothly. Or we pray with people for healing and they are healed. In short, we know we have the gift because the results are obvious.

Another way is when others point out to us that we have a gift in an area in which we did not think ourselves specially gifted. Many times, for instance, Emma Parent was told she made her guests feel especially welcome. A few out-of-town speakers our Institute brought in for conferences told me they had never been made to feel so much at home as when they stayed with Emma and her husband, Nelson. Emma had not previously thought she had the "gift of hospitality" (1 Peter 4:9), but she most certainly does.

Another way of discovery comes as we sense interest in a particular area of service. Often God will awaken an interest as a way of readying us for a gift He wishes to give us. I have watched several people who grew slowly but steadily in their ministries. It was quite clear: At one time they bore little fruit in a particular ministry and later they bore great fruit in it, but there was no one time when they took great jumps forward. God was raising their interest and slowly gifting them, testing their faithfulness and calling them progressively higher to greater usefulness (see Luke 19:16–17).

I should point out that just because we are interested in a particular ministry or sense we have a particular spiritual gift does not automatically mean we are called to that manner of service. I remember a man named Tim who thought he was gifted with the word of knowledge. In times of prayer with other members of a healing team, Tim would say regularly, "I believe God is telling me this or that" about a particular person on the team. Almost invariably Tim had it wrong. He was sincere, but he was sincerely mistaken. Because Tim was gentle in his approach and because he was among friends who understood the sometimes trial-and-error approach of discovering and using the spiritual gifts, no harm was done. But after several months of expressing what he thought were words from the Lord, Tim was finally persuaded that while God was gifting him in several things, the word of knowledge was not one of them!

The Gifts and Healing

Of the various spiritual gifts mentioned in Scripture, which come into play in the ministry of healing? In some ways they all do, although some more particularly so.

Gifts of healings

This is first and most obvious. The Bible does not speak of "a gift of healing," but of "gifts of healings" (1 Corinthians 12:28, NASB). It is a double plural. There is a variety of gifts in the ministry of healing and few persons, including those specially used in a healing ministry, seem to possess them all. We find that some have a particularly effective ministry to certain individuals—to children, for example—but not to everyone. Some exercise an effective healing ministry when an illness is related to a person's emotional distress, but not when it comes, say, from an injury. Some have success in praying for some illnesses but not for others. A person may have particular success in praying for asthma but not for cancer. I know someone who prays effectively for back problems but has little success in praying for headaches.

This does not mean that we should refuse to minister to those outside our area of chief effectiveness. If it seems, however, that God is using a particular person with great success in some aspects of the ministry of healing, we may want that person to pray for those whose problems fall into that area of ministry.

The word of knowledge

This is the gift of knowing a piece of information we have not learned or been told (1 Corinthians 12:8). It is something God tells us directly. The value of this gift is twofold. One, sometimes we do not know what particular problem is bothering an individual. Or if we do, we do not know its root cause. I recall counseling a man who seemed to be distressed but was not able to articulate what was troubling him. When I asked God silently to show me what the problem was, He revealed to me that the man was afraid his wife was being unfaithful. I asked the man gently if he was afraid his wife was having an affair. "Yes!" he blurted out. He was relieved that the concern was finally out on the table. Now, instead of chasing all around the barn in our conversation, we could focus on the problem.

It is not always necessary to know what the problem is. Sometimes it is sufficient to pray, "Lord, we lift Harry to Your throne of grace. You know what the need is." At other times it *is* important to know. The spiritual gift called the word of knowledge is useful at these times.

A second value of this gift is in demonstrating that God actually intervenes in lives today. A few years ago in St. Louis I was asked to pray for the sick in conjunction with a midweek service of holy Communion. About 25 people were present. As they remained at the altar rail after receiving Communion, I anointed each one with oil and prayed a brief prayer over each bowed head. Almost without thinking, I prayed a sentence like "Lord, please take away that anxiety" or "May her mother be healed of her gout" or "May that decision about the job be resolved."

After the service was over, they all waited to speak to me. One woman put it this way: "You don't know us or our problems. Yet as we discuss this among ourselves, we find that you prayed for specific problems in our lives and were correct every time. How did this happen?" I took that as an occasion to share, not only about the spiritual gifts, but about the reality, power and presence of God in the world today. One woman later commented to me privately, "My belief in God has always been fairly shallow. What happened today made me see that the things talked about in the Bible are real."

The word of wisdom

This is similar to the word of knowledge, except that "wisdom" is the specific application of truth to given situations (1 Corinthians 12:8). How often does someone know the truths of the faith but not how they apply to specific situations in life?

Sometimes this gift manifests itself in a regular, matter-of-course way. Some people are known for being wise. Whenever we face a dilemma or have to make a decision, they naturally share a wise piece of guidance with us. They have this gift, and are known for it.

Sometimes, however, this gift manifests itself in someone who does not have extraordinary wisdom, except on those occasions when God grants it. I mentioned Bertha earlier, the woman who lacks common sense but who can minister wisdom. I recall another situation in which a man on a healing team shared a helpful insight with a woman who had come forward for prayer. After she left our healing station, I asked Charlie how he knew what to tell her. "It had to be the Lord," Charlie replied. "I didn't know what I was saying until it came out. I felt as though God was giving me something to say. It certainly wasn't me!"

Prophecy

This means *forth*telling God's word in a particular situation (1 Corinthians 12:10). Prophecy is sometimes confused with "good preaching"; or preaching the Gospel as it relates to the sins of our day; or *fore*telling the future. Although a word of prophecy may involve all of these, the more precise definition of prophecy is God giving a specific word to a person or group via an individual. The word may come spontaneously at the time it is to be spoken, or God may give it ahead of time. It may be a word of comfort to those who are troubled, such as when God spoke about Israel in Isaiah 40:1. Other times it may be denunciation of sin, such as the Lord's rebuke of Israel in Amos 5:18–27. On far fewer occasions (and here it must be confirmed by other means of knowing God's will), it is a word of direction or guidance.

Let me give you an example of prophecy. I was the guest preacher one Sunday at a certain charismatic Episcopal parish. They had and still have an extensive ministry to the poor in their community. They seemed to be generous, giving folk. During a time in the worship service when the congregation was invited to speak any words the Lord was giving them, a visitor stood and said, "My children, you say that you love Me, but you are holding back. You must honor the poor in your midst. Do not reject them, for they are loved by Me."

Later I asked the woman who had given the prophecy why she said what she did. She told me she was mystified by those words. The congregation was one of the best examples she knew of a loving, caring ministry to street people. If anyone needed to hear that word, it wasn't *this* congregation. But she felt it was a prophetic word given to her by God and she had to speak it.

I asked the rector of the church what he thought. He told me it was right on target! Although the parishioners were involved in ministry to the poor, their attitude was one of charity, not love. The church ministered to the poor but saw them as *them*, and did not want *them* to be present for worship on Sundays. The prophetic word was God's way of saying that a change of attitude was sorely needed.

Since some of our physical and emotional sickness and much of our spiritual sickness is related to sin, a chastening word from God calling us to more righteous behavior relates to the ministry of healing. Additionally, as some of our emotional sickness and, therefore, some of our physical sickness can be traced to thoughts and feelings of worthlessness, a prophetic word of comfort relates to the ministry of healing.

It is imperative that any word claiming to be a word from God square with Scripture. God does not contradict Himself and will not give any word today that contradicts what He has given us once for all in the Bible.

It is also important to take seriously those prophetic words discerned to be authentic. Many churches tape-record at least that portion of the service during which people may bring forth prophetic words, or they have a team member write out any prophetic word given to an individual during times of ministry. Should the messages given during worship be deemed actual words from God, they are published in the Sunday bulletin the next week and the congregation exhorted to pay heed to them. The church leadership tries to discern what God would have the congregation do next, especially if several messages indicate a common theme.

Not every church is this responsible, however. I am familiar with more than one church proud of allowing prophetic words to be given in the Sunday service and during times of ministry, especially in contrast to other churches of the same denomination that are not open to the operation of spiritual gifts. I know one church that counts the number of different prophetic words it receives on Sunday but never seems to heed them. God does not send us words as toys or trophies but as tools—vehicles to bring us into greater conformity to God's will.

Speaking in tongues

Speaking in tongues is speaking a language we have not learned (1 Corinthians 12:10). Sometimes it is a known language, though not one known to the speaker. In his book *Nine O'Clock in the Morning,* Canon Dennis Bennett told how he tried in vain to minister to a man in the hospital. The man in the bed and Canon Bennett were unable to communicate because of a language barrier. Finally Canon Bennett started to pray over the man using the gift of tongues. While he did not know what he was saying, the man in the bed did. Later Canon Bennett discovered that he had been speaking a dialect of Spanish and that the words he spoke were a distinct blessing to the sick man.

The application to ministry should be obvious. Sometimes the barrier of human speech blocking effective ministry may be overcome through the gift of tongues. Such an experience, like the word of knowledge, demonstrates the reality of God.

A second way in which the gift of tongues is a blessing is as a personal prayer language. Scripture tells us that we do not always know how we should pray, so the Spirit helps us pray with sighs and groans too deep for words (Romans 8:26). I often have a burden to pray for someone or something. Using my prayer language (speaking in tongues as I pray), I feel the burden lift. I know God is providing the words. I may not know what I am saying, but God does.

Sometimes when I pray in this way I get a picture of or a thought about someone. On occasion I will be asked later, "Were you praying for me at such-and-such a time?" "Why, yes," I'll respond. "But I was praying in tongues so I don't know what I was praying for. Will you tell me?" Often they will, but more than once I have been told, "Oh, that's O.K. I would just as soon not have you know. The problem is resolved. I'm grateful you prayed for me. I'm also grateful God didn't tell you what the problem was!"

Mercy

This means giving mercy, comfort or compassion in a way far beyond what all Christians would normally give (Romans 12:8). This gift has great application to the ministry of healing. Sometimes what a person needs in order to be healed of emotional wounds is to receive genuine, deep love. At other times, as a person feels the mercy of another, he is able to share, perhaps for the first time, what his problems are. Once these are out in the open, other forms of ministry can help bring solutions. This can also enhance other forms of ministry. Confessing our sins, for example, works so much better when the confessor ministers in a merciful way. Many people find it far easier to deal with their sins with one who is understanding, not condemnatory.

Discernment of spirits

This is the gift of being able to know whether a person's underlying motive or the underlying power that controls a person is godly, human or satanic (Hebrews 5:14; 1 John 4:1). I recall praying with one man who was depressed. Depression can come from any number of root causes—seasonal adjustment disorder, hormonal problems, guilt over sins, hurt from being sinned against, false guilt feelings from Satan, an overly strict upbringing and so on. My attempts at ministering to this person had been unsuccessful and I was feeling frustrated.

A team member felt she was discerning a presence of evil hovering around the depressed person. She asked the man if he had been involved in occult practices. He responded that over the years he had been. For a while they had satisfied him, but eventually he stopped praying to God and attending church, and now he was feeling that the powers he had been calling on were turning against him. We led him in a prayer of renunciation of this involvement and within an hour the depression had lifted. It was not that *he* was evil, but that his involvement in the things of darkness, forbidden by God, had opened him up to evil spirits. The gift of discernment led my team member to know this.

Other gifts

Other spiritual gifts may not be as obviously related to the ministry of healing, but they do assist it. The gift of administration, for example, does not sound as though it relates to the ministry of healing, but consider how crucial to a large and active church-based healing team is a person with a gift for keeping things straight. Who but someone with administrative gifts (see 1 Corinthians 12:28) can keep track of the various requests for ministry, the team members who have the gifts needed for a particular person's need, and the making sure such ministry gets carried out? I know of one healing team in which one of the most valuable members is a person who never herself prays directly for the sick, but simply keeps track of those who do.

Using the Gifts in Ministry

Let me give you an illustration not only of how the gifts can be used in ministry, but how several spiritual gifts other than gifts of healings can come together.

Several years ago I was part of a four-person healing team at public services of healing. Let me give the names Ruth, John and Ida to the other team members. A man came to our prayer station at the front of the church. Even as he walked toward us, Ruth sensed within herself that this man, though appearing outwardly to be in fine shape, was hurting deeply. Ruth reached out her hands toward him and radiated the love and mercy of God. This enabled the man, whom I'll call Ed, to relax a bit and trust what we were doing.

Despite this, however, he was still unable to state his need. After a few moments of watching him struggle, John looked him right in the eye and said, "You're afraid your company will force you into retirement and you won't be able to provide for your family, aren't you?" Ed responded that this was indeed his concern, and he was glad John had said it because he knew he could not. The four of us prayed that God would work a miracle of some sort to help him in his circumstances. We prayed in addition that, whatever else happened, he would receive an emotional healing for the feelings of inadequacy and shame he was feeling, and that he would draw closer to God.

Then Ida, usually a quiet person, piped up, "I believe there are a few things you could be doing right now to help the situation and yourself." Ed listened to her suggestions and responded, "I've never thought of those things. But after hearing them, I believe you're right."

In that brief time of ministry several spiritual gifts came into play. First was the gift of knowledge, as God showed Ed's deep inner state to Ruth. Then came the gift of mercy as she offered God's tender comfort to someone in pain. John then manifested the gift of knowledge as he received supernatural revelation as to the nature of Ed's concern. Finally, Ida exhibited the gift of wisdom as she applied truths to a specific situation. No one was specifically used in a gift of healing *per se,* although the whole ministry taken together was therapeutic.

It is important to remember that using the various spiritual gifts requires both an empowering of the Spirit and a careful process of development. I have profited over the years from the phrase *fire in the fireplace.* It is from the book of the same title by Dr. Charles E. Hummel. I apply that phrase to the spiritual gifts in this way: If the various operations of the Holy Spirit, particularly the more spectacular ones, can be likened to a fire, and the careful, steady process of education, training and supervision to a fireplace, then the fire and the fireplace need each other.

We have all seen the harm done when one of these exists without the other. Fire outside the fireplace—the power and gifts of the Holy Spirit without proper safeguards—can become wildfire. It may be exciting and dramatic, but it can also burn down the house. As Victor Borge used to say, "My parents yelled at me for building a fire in the living room, probably because we didn't have a fireplace in the living room." When the spiritual gifts are not used wisely, people are not just warmed by the ministry of others, but fried to a crisp.

On the other hand, a beautiful fireplace may be aesthetically pleasing, but with no fire burning in it we are left cold and dark. Many churches that attempt to do ministry without seeking the empowerment of the Spirit and His gifts may have impressive programs and leaders with academic qualifications but leave people spiritually cold. We need to ask such churches the tough question of whether they see themselves as spiritual bodies or merely secular organizations with a veneer of religion. I know one priest, a fine man not as yet converted to Christ, who had the integrity to leave church work when he noticed that his people were no better for being members of a church than a similar number of unchurched people. Only after he was converted and filled with the Holy Spirit did he return to parish work. Now he sees lives being transformed on a regular basis. As Martin Luther wrote in his hymn "A Mighty Fortress Is Our God," "Did we in our own strength confide, Our striving would be losing."

Simply put, we need *both* the fire of the Spirit and the fireplace of education, training and supervision in ministry. This dual approach characterized Paul's guidance of his young protégé, Timothy. Paul told his young disciple, "Rekindle the gift of God that is within you through the laying on of my hands; for God [gave us] a spirit of power . . ." (2 Timothy 1:6–7). But he also told him, "Do your best to present yourself to God as one approved, a workman who has no need to be ashamed, rightly handling the word of truth" (2 Timothy 2:15). Rekindle the fire; be trained.

As for the fire, we pray and have others pray with us that God will empower us for service. We note that even Jesus did not begin His ministry until His human nature was filled with the Spirit at His baptism in the Jordan River. We ask God to give us the spiritual gifts He wants us to have. We do not rule out any of the gifts. We keep before us the truth that we cannot accomplish anything of lasting value by our own strength; otherwise we may grow luscious foliage but not fruit. Before we minister, we ask for divine protection, empowerment and guidance. After we minister, we ask for a refilling of the Holy Spirit and God's protection.

As for the fireplace, we read about wise, proper use of whatever gifts we have been given. We recall that not only have others in centuries gone by been used in the spiritual gifts, but they left behind wise words of caution, warning and guidance—words we neglect at our peril. We learn from those already ministering in an effective, balanced way. We submit ourselves to one another and to the leadership of our churches. We ask God to give us an attitude of humility, for the gifts are exactly that—gifts. They are not merit badges or accomplishments, nor are they rewards for being spiritually mature. The reason, I believe, that no one person has all the gifts of the Spirit (1 Corinthians 12:29–30) is that we will have to depend on one another as we depend on God.

As we minister we need to remember that we have this heavenly treasure in earthen vessels (2 Corinthians 4:7). As my friend Tim learned, a person does not always have the gifts he thinks he has. We can make mistakes. First Corinthians 13:12 tells us we know only in part. However much God may use us, we are still fallible creatures. This is why spiritual direction, supervision in ministry and accountability to others are so vitally important.

It is also why we need to be gentle. Using the gifts in an overly self-assured, high-powered way is wrong for several reasons. First, it scares people. People are so busy looking for the means to get away from someone ministering in this manner that they are not able to receive his or her ministry. Second, such a ministry is often done in human power rather than in the power of the Holy Spirit. Third, it often wrongly establishes superiority on the part of the one ministering and dependence on the part of the one receiving such "ministry." One is not taught to listen to the Holy Spirit for oneself but to keep going back to a person claiming a superior ability to hear God speak or minister God's blessings. Fourth, we might be wrong. The Bible tells us (as we just saw) that we know only in part. If we are proven wrong after having asserted that we know exactly what God is saying, people might be turned off to the subject of the spiritual gifts in particular or even to God Himself.

It is also important to understand that God can use people in the spiritual gifts at various levels. That is to say, one person may be used frequently in, let's say, the gift of knowledge, while another person may be used only occasionally. It has been my experience that when one or two members of a healing team are used regularly in a particular gift, the other members tend to rely on them too much for that kind of ministry.

The truth is that God can use any Christian who is open to Him, in any gift, at any time. While it seems that God *tends* to use certain people in certain gifts, we should not limit Him. We should never become too dependent on one or two people, therefore, but rather stay open to God, who surprises us with what He will do through each member of the team.

Similarly, we need to avoid seeing the spiritual gifts as our permanent possessions. God can cease to use us in particular gifts and start using us in others. Bishop Michael Baughen once said that as rector of a church in the English Midlands, his great gift was writing contemporary-style songs of praise, but when he moved to London to become rector of All Souls Church, Langham Place, his music-writing pen dried up and he wrote no more songs. Instead, he noticed that his ability to teach and preach increased significantly. Then, when he became bishop of Chester, God started using him in gifts more applicable to the office of bishop.

When we think of the gifts as our permanent possessions, we are in danger of being closed to God's future plans for us. In addition, we become proud, forgetting that the gifts are talents on loan from God.

As we realize that God has much work for His people to do and that we cannot do it without His empowering grace, we will see how important the spiritual gifts are for the work of ministry. We will understand that the spiritual gifts far transcend any particular theology of the Holy Spirit or cultural manifestation regarding them. We will know that the gifts are not just for some people but for all members of the Church to enable us to do the work God has given us, for the betterment of His people and the glory of His name.

Discussion Questions

1. Distinguish between natural talents and spiritual gifts.
2. What part do spiritual gifts play in the Body of Christ?
3. What is the significance of the double plural "gifts of healings"?
4. How do other spiritual gifts assist in healing?
5. Would it be appropriate to pray for a particular gift to assist your ministry in a particular situation? Discuss.
6. Name and describe three major objections to spiritual gifts.
7. What do you think 1 Corinthians 13:8–10 means by *when the perfect comes?*

Experiment

If you have not already done so, find out what your spiritual gifts are. List them in your notebook and do what is necessary to release them for ministry. Keep an accurate account of what you do and of what happens.

11

How to Introduce a Healing Ministry into Your Church

The point of studying Christian healing, of course, is so that you will, by God's grace, be able to minister to the sick in a sane, balanced and effective way. A hungry person, after all, does not want to learn about good cuisine; he wants to eat! We wish, similarly, to provide a vehicle whereby people may receive God's healing blessings. Our concern is to do the job and do it in such a way as to minimize the risk of causing disharmony and division. God calls us to dwell together in unity (Psalm 133:1; Ephesians 4:3) and to be at peace with one another (Mark 9:50; Romans 12:18). It would be tragically ironic to introduce healing into a church in such a way as to put the church into dis-ease. Dr. Peter Wagner underscored this in a humorous way when he entitled his book *How to Have a Healing Ministry Without Making Your Church Sick*.

Whenever a healing ministry is introduced in a church—or indeed, whenever any significant change is attempted—at least three different kinds of people emerge. You need to be aware of this and try to understand the thoughts, needs and

229

motives of these persons and respond to them wisely. If you do not, your healing ministry may never get going, and in some cases disaster can ensue!

The first kind of person might be called *the enthusiast.* Enthusiasts will want you to move the congregation into the ministry of healing at a rapid rate, whether the congregation is ready or not. Sometimes the enthusiast will try to convince you that anyone who does not become excited immediately about Christian healing must be a nonbeliever or else be harboring dark motives.

It is easy to be susceptible to enthusiasts: They seem to be our biggest supporters. They agree with what we are trying to do and they bring us encouragement and confidence when we are having doubts. But they can be harmful. Sometimes the enthusiasts scare away those who would have embraced Christian healing had they been allowed to do it at a more gradual pace. Sometimes the enthusiasts cause us to skip necessary steps in the planning or educational processes or to ignore issues in which prudent caution and regular supervision are needed.

How do you make use of the enthusiasm of these people while preventing the damage they can do? Try to channel their zeal into worthwhile projects. Try to keep them from occupying center stage in your endeavors, lest the ministry of healing be identified with them too closely in the minds of the congregation. If they are at all open and teachable, point out the need and reason for practicing patience and gentleness.

If these individuals are not tractable regarding their enthusiasm or if they show any other personality traits that could be harmful or disruptive to others, they need to be helped pastorally to discover the reasons for their behavior, and pray about and work on both the behavior and the root causes behind it. Such reactions indicate underlying problems of either a spiritual or emotional nature or both.

The second kind of person might be called *the honest doubter.* Honest doubters are open-minded people who often become supporters of the ministry of healing, *once they are convinced*. The idea of God's healing the sick in response to prayer is new to them. It sounds odd, quite possibly unscientific, even superstitious. It brings to mind those faith healing ministries that have gone wrong and brought hurt and division. The honest doubter would like to believe, but does not want anything for his church that is crazy or harmful.

Answer the questions of the honest doubter as best you can. (Chapter 3, "Objections and Answers to the Ministry of Christian Healing," will help.)

Genuinely thank the honest doubters for their concerns about what might go wrong. They may well be bringing godly wisdom. Encourage them to pray that only God's will be done.

The third kind of person is *the blocker*. Blockers may raise the same objections as honest doubters. The difference is, while honest doubters will come on board the ministry of healing once their objections are answered and their fears allayed, blockers do not want answers or assurance. They do not want this change—or often, any change—to take place. Sometimes it is insecurity that makes them cling to the past instead of to God. Sometimes they wish to maintain a tight control over what they regard as their personal fiefdom—their church. Sometimes they know instinctively that if God is at work healing, they will have to confront Him in a way that will demand commitment. On occasion blockers are "enemy agents" sent by the evil one to inhibit and prevent ministry.

Blockers may try devious ways to impede the ministry of healing, such as spreading malicious gossip or heightening fears that this is something bizarre. Perhaps, more subtly, they will raise concerns about people being hurt or turned off, or that the congregation isn't "ready" for this kind of ministry. Any pastor who is not careful could, out of love for the flock, become so susceptible to the fear of people's being hurt or offended that he would have nothing further to do with healing. When that happens, people will be hurt all the more, for they will miss out on a ministry that helps at the deepest levels of need. The pastor should listen lovingly to the concerns of the blockers, but not let them drag the healing ministry to a halt. Our marching orders for ministry come from what God tells us to do, *not* from those who are resistant to Him, no matter how important they seem to be or how much they pledge.

How to Proceed?

Given the fact that these three kinds of people may emerge as your church learns about a ministry of healing, how should the clergy and lay leadership proceed? Here are six areas of direction.

Study

In order to introduce the ministry of healing into a church, there needs first to be a well-thought-through period of education. The clergy and lay leadership would do well to plan a several months' or a year's program of education before embarking on a healing ministry. To those already convinced about healing, this may sound like a long time, but the rest of the church needs to be brought on board at the rate they can absorb this new information, especially if Christian healing seems radically different from what they have hitherto been taught.

We need to remember that the worldview of many in the Church is this-worldly and rationalistic. No matter how otherwise pious and devout, no matter how decent and moral, no matter how dedicated and active, many people simply do not believe that God intervenes directly in people's lives, nor do they have any evidence from their own experiences that He does. They have lived their lives with such a view for so long that it will take a while, often quite a while, for them to think otherwise.[1]

Let me illustrate how something that seems perfectly normal to one person may seem to another foreign to the point of being ridiculous. Several years ago on a ministry trip abroad, I spent some time in rural Kenya. Let's suppose I was speaking through an interpreter to a group of people in a remote tribal village about my years growing up outside of Boston. I might tell them of superhighways, trolley cars and subway trains. Generally speaking they could fit these modes of transportation into their frame of reference. While never actually having seen any of them, at least they do see the occasional Land Rover, and could extrapolate from that to other modes of transportation. What I said would be new but not ridiculous.

But what if I spoke to them about blizzards? How could these people, living in the tropics, possibly understand a three-day storm of bitter cold, howling winds and an accumulation of a white substance measuring 25 inches deep that lay on the ground for months afterward? A few people might believe me, especially if I had otherwise proven myself to them to be a decent, believable person. But many others might think I was speaking in myths—where the general point of the story is true but the details are not at all to be taken literally. Others might think I was trying to deceive them to gain money or power. Still others might think I had taken leave of my senses. In their frame of reference, how could accounts of a New England blizzard possibly be true?

In the same manner, how can church members who have been taught all their lives to believe that God does not intervene directly to change things come to believe that healings take place in answer to prayer? It would seem equally far-fetched. Thus, we have to educate people—carefully, thoroughly, patiently.

We need to set a context for what we are going to say. Lest the concept of healing look bizarre and foreign, we need to place it into the context of what people already know and accept. We do this in three ways.

First, we show how much the four Gospels deal with healing, and how healing both signifies and effects the inbreaking of the Kingdom of God. We compare healing with the resurrection: If God indeed raised Jesus Christ from the dead such events as healing in response to prayer are eminently possible.

Second, we encourage people to tell their own stories of times when God did something extraordinary in their lives in response to prayer. I believe that every church has people with stories to tell. Let me illustrate with two examples:

The first is about healing. I was filling in one Sunday for a priest who was ill. At the eight o'clock service I preached on healing and on how God still heals today. While shaking hands at the front door, I noticed one elderly woman lagging behind the rest. This often means a person has something to say but, for fear of embarrassment, wants to do it out of earshot of the others. Sure enough, in whispered tones she said to me, "I was dramatically healed once! It was thirty years ago when Agnes Sanford prayed for me." I asked her why we were whispering. She said, "No one here would believe me."

On the way back up the center aisle of the church, I spotted a woman in a pew who appeared to be kneeling in prayer. Actually, she was waiting for me and grabbed me as I went by. Again, in whispered tones, she told me she had been to a Roman Catholic shrine and was healed instantaneously of a medical problem. She told me, too, that the people in the church would laugh at her if she told her story.

Two more women spoke to me after the service telling me how they were healed in dramatic, noticeable, lasting ways. Each thought she was the only one in the church who had had such an experience, and that everyone else would laugh.

If only we could get people to tell their stories to each other! They would discover they were not alone and that, far from being ashamed for believing what the Scriptures teach about healing, they could share this good news with others confidently.

My second story builds on the first. I was an adjunct staff member for several years at St. Paul's Church in Malden,

Massachusetts. One day I was conducting a midweek noon Eucharist/healing service and preached on how some people today, as in Bible times, have been blessed to receive visitations from angels. I told those gathered that while this is not something that happens to everyone, nor should anyone think himself better for having received such a visitation nor worse for not having received one, these events sometimes happen today. After the service, while the dozen or so people were greeting each other, one woman shared that she had once seen an angel. A few others then shared their experiences, appreciative that they could tell someone else for the first time. Others expressed the fact that although this had never happened to them, they believed it did take place. One dear elderly lady said she would love to have an angel appear in her kitchen someday. This was the first time any of them had had the opportunity to share about this matter. It was a blessing for them to be able to do so, and a blessing for the others to hear the accounts.

My point is this: Many people have stories to tell. They need to tell them. Others need to hear them. When our stories are told in a gentle, humble manner, others are freed to tell their stories and to believe that God is working today in the lives of people like themselves. Thus they are encouraged to ask God for His help. Parishioners see that healings occur in churches like theirs, to people like themselves, in situations that are not bizarre. Sharing our stories "legitimizes" healing for many people: It is O.K. to pray for healing and expect God to go to work.

One man put it to me this way: "I never believed in all this stuff until it happened to my friend Jim. He had gone to a healing service for chronic back problems. He was prayed for and felt a tremendous sense of heat in his back at that time. He's been well ever since. I don't trust those frauds on TV, but I do trust Jim. He's convinced me this stuff about healing is for real."

Ask people to share their stories of healing before the congregation on Sunday, in a sharing group or on a special occasion. Or have them write out their stories and place them in the church newsletter or bulletin.

Another way to make use of healing testimonies is sharing with your congregation the stories of others. Ask the pastor of a nearby church if he has a parishioner who has a story to tell, and borrow that person. Make use of the testimonies of healing in Christian magazines. *Sharing* magazine of the Order of St. Luke is a good resource. It is devoted solely to Christian healing.

Three words of caution, however.

First, make sure that the people who share are ones who will add to the credibility of healing, not detract from it, and will keep the focus of their testimonies on God, not themselves or others. If a person rubs people the wrong way or is thought to be a fanatic or religious crackpot, his testimony of healing—however genuine—might have the opposite effect, alienating people from the ministry of healing, not drawing them to it.

Second, make sure that the testimonies of healing are not all of the dramatic, instantaneous variety. God heals in a variety of ways. We may keep people from receiving all God has in store for them if we are, in effect, encouraging them to believe He works only one way.

Third, set healing in a context by showing that your denomination believes in healing. Now, not everything one's church believes or has believed is true, of course. Churches err. But when a church's statement of faith and traditions are illustrative of biblical truth, we can make use of them to show it is O.K. for people in their denomination to believe in healing.

It would be humorous if it were not sad that some people do not care whether or not something is in the Bible as long as it is Methodist (or Baptist or Episcopalian, etc.). But until they come to trust the Scriptures as the primary authority for belief and practice, we can certainly remove roadblocks by showing how the healing ministry we want to introduce is part of our denomination's belief. We might call this the "kosher factor." Healing is "kosher" in our church—it is O.K. Episcopalians, for example, can point to the service of healing in *The Book of Common Prayer* and the reference to it in the Catechism. They can refer to the detailed and highly favorable report on Christian healing issued by the 1964 General Convention and subsequent statements since. They can point to the powerful healing ministries of Bishop William Cox in the United States and Bishop Morris Maddocks in England. People of other denominations can, to various degrees, do the same from the statements of faith, orders of services, denominational reports and statements of leaders of their churches. Confronted with all of this, no one whose concern is fidelity to the denominational heritage can oppose Christian healing. In fact, denominational loyalists, to be consistent, should *insist* that their churches have ministries of healing.

Thus, by placing healing in the context of what we already believe, we can make it much easier to introduce an intentional ministry of healing into a congregation.

The local church has various means at its disposal for educating its people about healing.

Sermons

In the course of the year, and especially during the time when the ministry of healing is being introduced, several sermons should be devoted to aspects of Christian healing. In addition to the pastor's teaching, other voices should be heard. Occasionally someone wonders why we devote several sermons to this one subject. The answer is, frankly, that we have to make up for years of no (or sometimes bad) preaching on the subject. In addition, a sermon is supposed to move people to action. It will take more than one sermon to move people to avail themselves of the ministry of healing and to seek God expectantly in prayer for His intervention.

The church newsletter

We have already seen that carefully selected testimonies of healing given by respected people in the congregation can have a salutary effect. A major article on Christian healing should appear in the newsletter from time to time. With permission, articles from Christian magazines can be reprinted. (Please be sure to secure permission. It is ironic that in the attempt to make the church more attuned to the blessings of God, some should violate the fundamental commandment not to steal!) Once again, this is not to be seen as a one-time event, but an ongoing educational process. In the months following a major article on healing, put in brief teachings of 75 to 150 words focusing on some aspect of healing. This serves to keep the topic in the forefront of parishioners' thoughts.

Adult education classes

Churches are increasingly rediscovering the truth that Christian education is for people of all ages. Many churches have adult education hours before, after or between Sunday services. Many churches have a weeknight forum or study group. A segment of several weeks can be devoted to Christian healing. Participants can read and discuss books. They can listen to video or audio tapes. (The Institute for Christian Renewal has available a wealth of resources on Christian healing; see p. 357.) In your study materials do not neglect the scriptural accounts of healings performed in the Old Testament, by our Lord and by the early Christians. (A list of these appears in Appendix 3.)

Speakers

An outside speaker can be brought in for a weekend healing mission. A three-day healing mission might look something like this:

Friday evening: Covered-dish supper followed by a general, introductory overview of Christian healing. The nature of this program generally draws a good percentage of the committed members of the congregation. You may wish to invite people from other churches or the general public or else you may wish to concentrate on members of your own congregation. The second option may be especially wise if this is your church's first large-scale introduction to healing.

Saturday: Further teaching on various aspects of Christian healing. This session generally draws only those truly committed to Christian healing, especially those who will likely form the parish healing team. It is not unwise to have such concentrated teaching for those who eventually will be doing the ministry.

Saturday evening: Either a healing service open to the public with members of the parish healing team assisting (even if this is their very first time praying for the sick), or an informal gathering in a parishioner's home to discuss practical ways of implementing or enhancing a church-based healing ministry. This may be the better choice if it seems to be too soon for a public healing service, or if the perceived need is to develop a strategy. If this is your choice for Saturday evening, it is important to have present both those who would like to be part of the ministry of healing and those in positions of authority, leadership and decision-making.

Sunday morning: A simple, basic message on healing as the sermon. While this may be anticlimactic for those who have participated fully in the weekend, it is important to get the rest of the congregation on board, many of whom were not at any sessions of the weekend's mission. You may wish to have a carefully selected testimony of healing given. Sometimes it is appropriate for people to be invited to the front for healing prayer.

I have been asked why I recommend a weekend-long special emphasis on healing. The answer is this: We put special emphasis from time to time on different aspects of our faith.

There are times, for example, when we place special emphasis on stewardship. We do not think good stewardship is less important on other occasions, of course, but we do call special attention to this aspect of Christian discipleship from time to time. Similarly, many churches have a time in the course of the year when special emphasis is put on Christian education, social responsibility, foreign missions, repentance (especially during Lent) and so on. So, too, with healing. But, just as with these other aspects of the faith, highlighting healing on particular occasions does not mean to imply it is not part of the regular, ongoing life of the church.

The example of the clergy and others who believe in healing

If the clergy have taught about healing but respond to someone's illness with sympathy and the telephone number of a specialist, not with an offer to pray for healing, they are saying by their actions that Christian healing is not real. It is something to talk about, in other words, but not to believe in. If, however, the clergy respond to sickness with immediate, believing prayer (and perhaps also anointing with oil), they are saying that they truly believe healing works. I observed one church that came to believe in and experience God's healing through prayer because of the regular, gentle ministry of an elderly assistant pastor who visited people at home and in the hospital, sharing scriptural truths and his personal experience of healing, praying with them for God to intervene.

In like manner, when one who claims to believe in healing asks others to pray for him when he falls sick, he is demonstrating that he really believes his words. This may sound silly to some, but large numbers of people do think that church people in general and clergy in particular are supposed to say certain things that they do not, in fact, believe in.

In the sixfold manner described above, a regular, systematic, ongoing method of education about healing will answer questions, defuse objections, raise hope and give careful instruction about the ministry of healing you are anticipating.

Services of Healing

In addition to the ministry of healing conducted in the context of visits to people in the hospital or in their homes, public services of healing are ways in which our Lord's healing is made available to His people. Here are three different times at which you may wish to have such services:

Daytime, midweek

Have prayers for healing, the laying on of hands and anointing of individuals in the context of a daytime midweek Communion service. The advantage of this kind of service is that it makes the healing ministry available to those, especially the elderly, who cannot come out at night. Although in many churches this is the only time intentional prayers for the sick are offered, it has the disadvantage of being inaccessible to most people. We need, therefore, to provide healing prayer at other times as well.

Evening—midweek or Sunday

There are two ways to have evening services:
One, a program or service where healing ministry is available but is not the main focus of the evening. Many churches have midweek or Sunday evening services of prayer and praise, adult Bible studies or fellowship. Healing prayers and anointing can be made available in the course of the evening's event, or after the event for those who wish to stay.

Two, a service of healing *per se,* in which the whole service is oriented around healing, with hymns, Scripture readings, personal testimonies, teaching and prayers on the theme of healing. Prayers for individuals with laying on of hands and anointing with oil could be placed after the sermon, right after Communion is taken or after the final blessing/dismissal. There are advantages to each of these three approaches:

After the sermon. If the sermon is an encouragement to faith in the God who expresses His inexhaustible love through healing (among other ways), having healing prayers directly after the sermon gives people an opportunity to respond while the thought is fresh in their minds.

After receiving Communion. In the early centuries of the Church, Communion was seen as a sacrament of healing. In the course of preparing to receive Communion, we have confessed our sins (often necessary to remove a blockage to healing), focused on our Lord's self-giving love in dying for our sins, and knelt in humility and anticipation. In receiving Communion we receive Him into our lives in a special way and receive His grace. To proceed directly from receiving Communion to receiving healing prayer adds to—and in many cases completes—the process of healing.

After the service is over. An advantage here is that the team can take more time with individuals. This is especially significant once the number of people requesting prayer grows to more than two dozen. Although God can, and often does, heal in response to a one-sentence prayer, sometimes it is more helpful to have soaking prayer—that is to say, prayer that soaks in gently over a longer period of time. Sometimes words of counsel from the team members, a time of sharing or asking for guidance or a period of confessing of sin is needed. Sometimes the person we are praying for loses composure and needs time to regain it. Sometimes the therapeutic value of spending time with people who obviously need our loving presence is most helpful. By delaying the time of prayer until after the service is over, the tendency to rush is lessened. Those who need to leave can do so without embarrassment. Our tendency to pray too quickly, as we notice how long things are taking, is dealt with, for people are free to leave when they wish.

There are a few disadvantages to delaying prayer ministry until right after the service. The people who are helped do not have the immediate opportunity to share with the rest of the congregation. Thus an opportunity to give glory to God is lost, as is the opportunity to strengthen the faith of those not yet prayed for. The added power of a larger number of people either praising God in song or praying from the pews for the healing ministry taking place up front is seriously diminished.

I have made use of each of the three times of offering healing ministry in an evening service and find that each has its advantages. The healing team should both discern prayerfully and monitor carefully to see which seems to be best at a given time.

Sunday morning

There is much to be said for having healing available every Sunday in conjunction with the services of worship.

Theologically, it demonstrates graphically the truth that the God we worship cares and wishes to meet us at our points of need. We would deem it foolish if a salesperson spent time articulating the various virtues of a given product only to fail to offer us the chance to buy. Yet in many churches, while the hymns, readings, sermon and prayers all speak of how God cares for us today, there is no direct opportunity for people to be brought to the throne of grace to receive the expression of such divine care.

Some object that because God knows a person's needs, such direct ministry is unnecessary. I tell them that God similarly knows our need for enlightening and motivation to do His will, yet we still preach sermons. Why have sermons, prayers, counseling or the sacraments if God's knowledge of our needs means that no direct action on the part of the Church is necessary? If we truly grasp how much God cares for hurting people and how much time Jesus spent ministering to them, if we understand how much healing has historically been a part of the Church, then we will find a Sunday service that lacks prayers for healing just as odd as we would a Sunday service that lacks prayer, Scripture, a sermon or a collection!

Practically, Sunday morning is the time when the largest number of our congregation is present. We appreciate physicians or government agencies that offer Saturday or evening hours, as it makes services more accessible. Should we not make the richness of God similarly accessible, especially when not everyone is convinced that healing works? In other words, parishioners who are "open but not yet convinced" might avail themselves of the ministry if it were offered on Sunday while they are already at church, but might not come to a midweek healing service. We hope they will eventually see the reality and power of such a ministry. But for now we have to start where they are; otherwise we may not get any further with them.

The question again arises as to where prayers for healing should be placed. As with a midweek service, there are three possibilities: after the sermon, after receiving Communion and after the service.

After the sermon. Some churches offer a litany of healing and a time of general prayer for categories of illnesses said for the congregation en masse, with pauses so individuals can add their own personal needs, silently or aloud.

Some churches deploy several teams of healing ministries in different locations around the church. People who want prayer would go to the team of their choice, state their concern in one or two sentences and receive a brief prayer (and anointing). The whole operation lasts no more than a minute per person. (If a person needs counseling, confession, inner healing, guidance, etc., he can be asked to meet with the team for further ministry after the service, or meet for the purpose of making an appointment for later.)

Other churches ask the congregation to break into groups of four or five right where they are in the pews. People then share their needs briefly and pray with and for one another. Some might object that this forces people to talk with each other, get involved in the hurts of others and engage in ministry themselves rather than leave it to the clergy and a few designated laypeople. To this objection I would say, "Yes! Exactly so!" Whatever one's style or preference of spirituality, Christianity is not a spectator sport; nor is it individualistic, sealed off from the lives and problems of others; nor is it done by a designated few for my benefit without my having to get dirty. While it may take some time to learn how to be a ministering community, the march toward that goal must not stop.

After Communion. The healing team receives Communion first, then proceeds directly to a side chapel or to an out-of-the-way section of the main church, or (as a last resort) to a special prayer room somewhere in the church building. An individual desiring ministry would go there right after receiving Communion. Those awaiting their turn for ministry would sit in a nearby pew ready to go to the next available ministry team, yet remaining enough distance away from the team to afford privacy and respect to the person to whom ministry is currently being directed. Done this way, there is no break between receiving Communion and receiving healing prayer (or prayerfully awaiting it). The service of worship continues and concludes while the healing ministry proceeds in its location.

After the service is over. The ministry begins right after the service is over. As others are either shaking hands at the door or proceeding to fellowship hour, those desiring prayer move to the front of the church. They remain in prayer near—but not too near—where the ministry is taking place, awaiting their turn. Churches with altar rails will find their use an advantage here.

Style

In most cases, the style of healing services should be in the
style of your church in general. Sometimes what turns people
off to the ministry of healing is not healing itself, but the style
in which it is expressed or the atmosphere that surrounds it.
If, for example, in a church whose worship style is gentle and
quiet, a healing service is conducted in the style of an ener-
getic revival meeting, the people of that church will have an
additional stumblingblock to overcome in their acceptance
of healing. If they see that healing can be ministered in a gentle, quiet style, however, this roadblock is removed.

Part of the problem comes from the fact that often those
most interested in establishing a ministry of healing have seen
it only in churches of a very different style. It is natural to
assume in those cases that this is the *only* way healing ministry can be conducted. In assuming this, however, substance
is confused with style—an easy thing to do. In order to prevent this from happening, we need to do four things.

First, remember how easy it is to fall into the trap of impos-
ing a foreign pattern onto your congregation and be on your
guard against doing that. This is not to say that God may not
be leading your church to move into different patterns of
worship. But doing that while introducing the healing ministry throws too much change at people at once and leads
them to link healing with the other changes. If they do not
like the other changes, they will assume it is the fault of the
healing ministry and reject it along with the other changes.

Second, remember that basic truths can be expressed in
different ways. I find it helpful to recall how different the
apostles were in personality—the blue-collar, rough-and-tum-
ble Peter; the intellectual yet emotional Paul; the serene, mystical John—yet how united they were in the faith and in commitment to Jesus. Try to imagine a "Peter kind of healing
service" or a "Paul kind" or a "John kind." I am sure they
would look very different, yet be equally effective.

Third, try to find a church similar to your own in style that has an effective healing ministry. Although you will not want to copy slavishly everything they do, chances are you will find that their experience and their way of prayer, worship and seeking God's blessings are what you are looking for.

Fourth, keep listening to the Holy Spirit to guide you. God knows what He wants for your church and will lead you into a format and style that are right for you. Remember, though, to keep listening. God will not keep things static. Our Friday night service in Malden took several different shapes over the years.

Supervision

You heighten significantly the chances of the acceptance of a healing ministry if you exercise careful supervision. Although God does not want a church's leadership to control—that's God's job—He does ask the leadership to be responsible for supervising what goes on.

You need to start by supervising the entire process of introducing the healing ministry to the congregation. It has been my experience that the way in which change is introduced has as much to do with its ultimate acceptance as the particular change itself. It is one thing for a minister to say, in effect, to a congregation, "We're going to have a healing ministry here. It's what God wants. So there!" It is an altogether different thing to say, "I'd very much like to have a ministry of healing at our church. After a period of teaching about it, I'd like a six-month experiment. During that time we'll watch carefully how it goes. If you have any questions, I'll answer them as best I can. I'd like your input and feedback. Then, after the experiment is over, let's stop and evaluate to see whether we should continue, and, if so, with what changes." Only the most negative, controlling or fearful person would oppose an honest and humble request like that.

In addition to the supervision by the pastor and congregation, it is wise to ask for a critique by an outsider experienced in the ministry of healing. He or she can bring both the wisdom that comes from experience, and the different perspective of an outsider.

As you introduce the ministry of healing, it is important to remember the scriptural admonition not to despise the day of small beginnings (see Zechariah 4:10). You are (or should be) building for the long term. It is better to build slowly and have something that lasts than to build quickly and see your work crumble and God's people alienated from the ministry of healing. In our admiration for the great, well-known ministers of healing, we often forget that many of them spent years in quiet obscurity, with little fanfare and with few people presenting themselves for prayer. Only after some long periods of testing and learning did these ministries grow.

We should not take "slow and careful" to mean "not at all." This ministry is too important to let our fears and cautions keep us from acting. But God's people must always remember the scriptural truth that "he who believes will not be in haste" (Isaiah 28:16).

You also need to exercise careful supervision of those who will compose the healing team. We will look at that more thoroughly in the next chapter.

Discussion Questions

1. Describe the good and bad aspects of each of the three kinds of people who surface when a healing ministry is proposed in a local church.
2. How can effective study of the subject of Christian healing occur?
3. What are the essential ingredients in beginning services of healing in a local church?

Experiment

Since this is necessarily a corporate function, and the experiment will have a profound effect, one way or the other, begin where you are, with as many others as are willing, toward a ministry of healing in your church. Include a prayer for wisdom every time you pray. Using this book, start moving cautiously and prayerfully from where you are to where God leads you. This experiment is the most important one. Record every step in your healing notebook.

12

The Selection, Training and Supervision of the Healing Team

Although it is true that God can use any believer to pray for the sick (Mark 16:17–18), much of the ministry of healing in a congregation will be conducted by the healing team. There is a reason for this. While divine call and Spirit empowerment are essential for ministry, so are careful training and supervision. The Lord Jesus spent three years training His closest followers carefully for the work they would do after He ascended to heaven. Paul told Timothy to study to show himself approved as a worker for God (2 Timothy 2:15). The parish healing team is a group of people like the apostles and Timothy who receive in-depth training and supervision, in this case for the ministry of praying for the sick.

It is not a good idea to ask for volunteers for this ministry because sometimes the wrong people step forward. Rather, we approach people we believe would make good ministers of healing and pray with them to see if they also perceive a call to this form of Christian service.

250

Qualities

Here are the qualities I look for in a minister of healing (or, indeed, in anyone who ministers to others):

Spiritual life

Remember, healing is not just the elimination of a physical or emotional problem. Healing is wholeness, and it comes, in part, as one grows into fuller stature in Christ. To help others come to that, the minister of healing needs to have a living, dynamic relationship with God in Christ. In addition, he or she should be working actively toward spiritual maturity.

Love of people

Many medical professionals are of the belief that patients recover more quickly when they have doctors who love them and are genuinely concerned for them as people. Anyone seeking prayer can soon tell whether or not ministry is being done out of genuine love and concern. (See what Jesus said about that in John 10:7–15.)

Ability to take direction

The pastor or healing team leader will sometimes ask a team member to minister or not to minister to a particular individual, or to do or not to do something as he or she ministers. There is not always time to give an explanation. On other occasions, because of issues of confidentiality, the leaders cannot give an explanation. At those times the team member must simply follow direction without argument. While no one is to follow an order involving something illegal, immoral or heretical, of course, on all other occasions the minister of healing is simply to obey.

A generally healthy emotional life

While we never outgrow our need for further emotional and spiritual healing—we are all, to use Henri Nouwen's phrase, "wounded healers"—a certain degree of emotional health is necessary in order to minister to others. If a person's need for succor is too high, the focus of his ministry will be his own needs, not the needs of others. If a person is ministering primarily to shore up a weak self-esteem, to look important to others or to gain favor with God, it is unlikely that he will offer the kind of ministry a hurting person needs. In fact, real harm can happen. Thus, we seek only those who have a generally healthy emotional life and self-image.

Teachability

We all have much to learn. Those people who are good candidates for membership on the team are the ones who can be corrected without getting hurt or angry. It is understandable for beginners in the ministry to make lots of mistakes. It is not acceptable for them to continue making the same mistakes because they refuse to be taught or corrected.

A desire to improve as a minister of healing

While the word *professionalism* carries some connotations inappropriate for Christian ministry, still, those involved are to take seriously the importance of being the best ministers of healing they can be. Just as physicians, teachers and musicians—to name just a few—should keep working to improve, so should those ministering healing. It is an important service. We want on our team, therefore, the kind of person who regularly rereads the accounts of healing in the New Testament, reads books about healing, goes to conferences on healing, seeks individual supervision, shares with others involved in the ministry of healing and so on. Some "jobs" around the church can be done by people with relatively low commitment or sluggish spiritual lives. Healing is not one of them.

What about people who offer themselves for the team who fall far short of these six criteria? We would be doing them a disservice if we, out of misplaced love or affirmation, put such people onto the team. Much experience has shown the damage that can ensue—harm to those who ask for healing and to the reputation of the healing ministry. While we are not to invite them onto the team, we are not simply to turn them away, either. They desire a good thing, however troubled they may be personally, or however confused they are in their motives.

I have told such people that I really appreciate their offer to help, and that, indeed, they may eventually be able to do fine ministry in healing, *but not right now.* I tell them that I would like to work with them on those things that are holding them back, to bring them, possibly, to a place where they would be ready to serve. I make them no promises for future healing team membership, but I do offer my help to assist them in their own healing and growth.

Some people have reacted to my offer with inappropriate hurt or anger, thereby demonstrating a problem area. Others have accepted the offer of help. It was, in some cases, the occasion of reaching them when before I had not been able to find a way. After various lengths of time, some of them grew to the point that it was appropriate for me to invite them onto the team. Their struggles with personal issues made most of them highly sensitive and most effective in their ministry to others.

You may have noticed that I did not list a "gift of healing" as one of the main criteria for selection. At the initial stage of team formation, this is not as crucial as the other criteria. God can still use these people in healing, of course, simply because they are believers. And often, with the humble service they are offering and their desire to grow, God will say to them, "Friend, come up higher. You have proven faithful in small things. I will now gift you in healing, that you may prove faithful over larger things."

Part of the reason we do not select only those with demonstrated gifts of healing for the team is this: How would we necessarily know who they are unless they are already ministering healing? In most churches, unless they are on a heal-

ing team, there is little opportunity for them to minister healing and thus demonstrate their gift. To cut through this
"Which came first, the chicken or the egg?" dilemma, we do
not base a person's selection on the demonstration of a
1 Corinthians 12 spiritual gift of healing but on a Mark 16:18
promise that God can use any believer, at least to some
degree, in healing.

I suggest that your initial team membership number
between four and eight people. More may well be ready, particularly in larger congregations. But since much of a team
member's initial training is one-on-one supervision, four to
eight is about all a supervisor will be able to handle effectively. After several months to a year of working with them
in their apprenticeship, they will be far enough advanced not
to need supervision of such a close variety. At that time you
can take a second group and work intensely with them, making use of people from the first group to help.

Training the Healing Team

Once you have selected the initial team, how do you go
about training them? You need to do three things.

Study

Building on the general congregational study of healing
already mentioned, much more learning is to be done. First,
do a careful study of each of the healings Jesus performed. (A
list of these appears in Appendix 3.) Do an inductive study of
each account of healing, bringing to each passage various questions. In its training course for new members, the Order of
St. Luke directs people to ask several questions about each
Scripture passage. (These questions are listed in Appendix 4.)

Going through each healing account to find the answers
to these questions is important. No matter how good the
books and tapes of the experts on healing are, our primary
source must always be the Scriptures. Have each person go

through the passages on healing individually, writing out the answers to the questions. Then get them together to share what they discovered.

Once this inductive study of Scripture is completed, do a systematic, topical study of the ministry of healing. You can do this by reading the earlier chapters of this book aloud in the group, by using other books or by listening to a series of teaching tapes on healing. (A bibliography is provided at the end of this book.) Periodically the leader should stop to make sure people understand what they are reading or hearing. The leader should formulate discussion questions about the material and pose them to the group. Some of the material covered may be review and some of it may be too advanced for immediate implementation. In any case, it is wise at this stage to get a big-picture overview of the subject.

Spiritual direction

In some churches this is called "discipling." Each member of the healing team should start meeting with a spiritual director on a regular basis. Spiritual direction is one of those marvelous things God has given to the Church. It almost died out at one point, but is now making a strong comeback. Spiritual direction is not to be confused with teaching, counseling, confessing sins or training for ministry, although it involves aspects of all of these. Rather, spiritual direction is assistance to help us reflect on and grow in our walk with God. The spiritual director helps us examine our prayer life so it can be improved. The director will talk with us about our struggles with temptation and sin, about our sensing (or not sensing) God's presence in our lives, about our hearing (or not hearing) God speaking to us and about how and in what ways we are sensing God at work in us and through us. We might describe a spiritual director as a coach of the soul, whose task is to help us grow in our personal relationship with God. Good teachers can help us intellectually; good enablers can help us functionally; good counselors can help us emotionally; but a good spiritual director helps us spiritually, in the narrow, technical sense of that word.

The criteria for a spiritual director include the various qualifications of a good confessor described previously (see pages 103–105), with one addition: a giftedness in guiding the growth of one's personal relationship with God. Some wise, godly people make wonderful teachers, confessors or preachers, but not necessarily good spiritual directors. In your quest to find one, ask the people you know who are particularly godly if they have a spiritual director and if you might contact him or her. Their spiritual director may be able to become yours as well. If not, he or she would likely be able to recommend someone. Make certain that the person to whom you are entrusting the care of your soul is spiritually mature and theologically orthodox. Ask questions of the person you feel might become your spiritual director and check him or her out with others whom you respect. Many people attempt to pass themselves off as spiritual directors when they really have no business doing so.

You may find, after several sessions with your spiritual director, that while this person may be a good spiritual director in general, he or she is not right for you. Perhaps your personalities do not mesh. Possibly the director is not knowledgeable in the area where you especially need guidance. Or there may be other reasons. If your spiritual director does not seem right for you, try another. Spiritual directors understand the need for directees to make a change. Make sure, however, that the reason you are changing directors is not because your director has zeroed in on issues with which you do not wish to deal.

If your spiritual director is not your pastor, the two should be in occasional contact. This is not to find out the details of what was discussed. If that were so, few people would talk with the candor necessary for adequate direction. Rather, it is so your pastor will be certain you are making the regular, good-faith effort at direction necessary for anyone rendering ministry, and so that he will be able to assist in your spiritual growth.

Why is spiritual direction so important? For one reason, a ministry of wholeness centers, as we have seen, in a personal relationship with God. If you are to help others come more fully into wholeness, the matter of your own personal wholeness is key. If your spiritual journey is not progressing, you need someone to help you discover why it is not. If it is growing, but in an eccentric way, you need assistance in discerning how to refocus it. Even if it is going well, you need someone to help you keep it that way.

As you pray with others, you may become aware of God speaking to you, perhaps in an unfamiliar way. You may sense God's presence, or believe Him to be absent. You may experience a spiritual "high" or what some have called "the dark night of the soul." In any case, ministry opens up new vistas in your relationship with God. If you are to take advantage of these opportunities, you need the wisdom of a wise spiritual coach.

Second, the task of ministry makes you vulnerable. The devil is threatened by Christians growing spiritually and bearing good fruit in ministry. He will try to attack you in various ways. He will send you various temptations, will seek to make you lazy, discouraged, proud, will put in your mind dark and lurid thoughts or will so stir up unresolved issues in your life that your focus will become yourself and not God and His work. A good spiritual director will bring you gentle comfort, loving reassurance and practical help when you are assaulted by the evil one.

Supervision

When people ask for prayers for healing, they are often at their most vulnerable. Something is wrong in their lives, or in the life of someone they love. As a result, they are more

likely at this time than at any other to be wounded by someone ministering in a careless manner. For this reason, many
people who believe in healing and have spent time studying
it are reluctant to pray for the sick. While they see the need,
they are afraid of hurting the very people they want to help.
Such caution is not only understandable, it is very wise. With
careful supervision, however, they can render ministry that
both gives help and avoids harm.

Two essential components to supervision, I believe, make
it likely that a new team member will render sound ministry.

The **first** is for the apprentice not to minister alone but
with someone experienced in ministry. (If the pastor perceives
the need for supervision in beginning a ministry of healing,
someone from another healing team may be borrowed for a
while.) The one experienced in praying for the sick offers
prayer while the apprentice watches and prays silently. After a
while, the apprentice takes the lead while the supervisor
watches (while also praying quietly). When ministry is done
this way, the apprentice can take those tentative first steps in
ministering knowing that someone more experienced will
intervene if the apprentice forgets what to say, offers inappropriate ministry or if something should go wrong.

Second, after the service is over, the supervisor reviews
what the team member has done in ministering. This review
session will usually be brief, as the team has spent quite some
time praying before the service, and attending and ministering at the service itself. More extensive review occurs later.
This review can take place in either a one-on-one session, at
a team meeting or, preferably, in both. Several kinds of issues
are discussed.

The Issues in Review

Theological issues

Several theological issues are raised when one is ministering, such as: "Why is this person suffering? He seems to be

such a fine man." "When prayer was being offered, I felt heat in my hands [or heat coming from a certain place on the sick person's body]. What does this mean?" "I didn't see anything happen. Is this ministry real?" These and other questions may arise in the mind of the apprentice. They may also be asked by the person for whom we are praying. Having done our introductory studies in Scripture and in books and tapes, we now go back to the sources for answers to these questions. Theology, which can be dry when done by itself, now takes on life and meaning when we see its relevance to the questions that come up.

Practical issues

When one does ministry, all sorts of practical questions arise, such as: "What do I do if someone starts crying?" "If I believe that her need is other than, or in addition to, the one she stated, do I pray for that, too, and if so, how?" "If the power of the Holy Spirit comes down in such a way that the person for whom we are praying is noticeably affected, what do we do?" "If I'm in the hospital praying and the doctor or nurse comes in, how do I explain what I'm doing and ask them to give us a few minutes?"

Questions always come up regarding confidentiality. How much do we tell our supervisor? If he or she happened to be present when the ministry took place, there is, of course, no problem. But if we are reporting on something that took place when our supervisor was not there, how do we get the critiquing necessary for our growth as ministers of healing, while respecting the confidentiality of the ones ministered to? There are two ways.

One is to change the superficial, irrelevant details of the story as we share it. This disguises the identity of the individual. If we are presenting for supervision the case of a 28-year-old businessman from our church, for example, we could change it to a 54-year-old housewife whom we know in a social context. There are two occasions, however, in which this will not work. One is if those details are germane to the situation. Some stories cannot be reworded to protect confidentiality without making the feedback we need off-target. The other—much more common, especially in small churches—is that no matter how we change the details, people know whom we mean.

The other way is to ask the person's permission. If we tell the person that we, for the purpose of our own growth and for the sake of those we will minister to in the future, need to discuss the case with the person supervising us, permission is often given. Many times, when we need to present a case to the whole team, the matter for which we are praying is not particularly embarrassing and permission will be readily forthcoming. If we are unable to get permission to share one particular case with the group, we may be able to get permission for another one.

Personal issues

As we minister, we get in touch with unresolved hurts or guilt from the depths of our own souls. As for hurts, I remember praying with another person for a man whose son had drowned in a swimming pool accident. No sooner did he tell us his story than my prayer partner burst into tears. She, too, had lost a son in an accident. She thought she had worked through her loss adequately, but it became apparent that more grief work was necessary.

As for guilt, the request that a group of us pray for a man dying of liver cancer raised guilt feelings in one of the members of the team. She wondered if she had done enough to pray for and visit her grandmother when she was dying of cancer.

In both cases, being involved in ministry brought to the surface issues that had been either repressed or ignored. They became the focus of supervisory sessions. In both cases, the individuals involved were grateful that those matters were identified so that they could be resolved. We should be aware that when we are ministering, many such issues will come to the surface. While this may be distressing emotionally, it is a wonderful opportunity to address and resolve those matters that, while not conscious to us, nevertheless do us harm.

Spiritual issues

Because the ministry of healing is just that—a ministry—it does not leave us unaffected spiritually. How do we discern the voice of God from other voices speaking to us? Is what I am experiencing a gift of the Holy Spirit, and if it is, how do I use this gift? What is God teaching me about Himself and myself in this? How do I deal with the personal, spiritual issues that are arising in me? Such issues might include an awareness of my need to pray better and more often, a conviction of a particular sin, a new awareness of God and so on. Because theological, practical, personal and spiritual issues are all interconnected, they should be raised in supervisory sessions even though we will also discuss them with our spiritual directors.

At first we may be surprised at how many things there are to discuss. It must be for this reason that God blesses the new team member with only a few people seeking prayer. Much time is needed at the beginning to address the various issues that ministry raises. I remember talking with several people who were disappointed that their services of healing attracted only a few people. I was able to convince them that each person prayed for raises a whole number of questions that the team would be wise to address. I have seen ministries of healing go very wrong because time was not spent at the beginning doing the careful reflection necessary. (I have listed some questions for review in Appendix 9, "Case Study Review Questions.")

I have also heard from people how the time of apprenticeship became the time when they grew the most spiritually. One woman put it this way: "My prayer life and reading of Scripture took on an urgency, as did the resolving of various personal issues in my life. In order to help people, I had to take my walk with God seriously. I was forced to grow up spiritually, and I did!"

While some of the healing team may always be "general practitioners," others may sense a calling or find a particular giftedness in ministering to one kind of person, in using particular gifts of the Spirit or in one sub-specialty of healing. In those cases we will encourage them to further prayer, reading and even apprenticeship to a person with a recognized, effective and balanced ministry in that particular aspect of Christian healing.

Deploying the Team

A healing team can be deployed in several ways. We'll look at three of them.

Hospital or home visitation

Two team people (any more than two quickly tires the person being visited) visit a sick person "on location" and pray for the specific problems. They must remember that while friendly chitchat is certainly welcome, the main purpose of the visit is prayer, so that, by the grace of God, the sick person will improve in health and be drawn closer to God. They should also remember that anyone sick enough to be housebound or hospitalized has a limited amount of strength. The tone should be gentle. The visit should be brief.

Wise is the pastor who takes along his apprentices when making such visits. Not only are there more people praying, but the apprentices have the chance to learn by observation and supervised participation.

Altar rail ministry

In a growing number of churches, healing prayer is offered at a prayer station in one corner of the church, in a side chapel or in a separate room. This ministry (as I mentioned earlier) is brief, no longer than a few minutes per person. The person desiring prayer states his or her concerns in a sentence or two, and the members of the team respond. While the problem is being presented, the team members engage in what is called active listening—that is, listening carefully to make sure not only that they have gotten the surface details correct, but that they are perceiving any underlying patterns. They ask God quietly for wisdom on how to proceed.

Team members lay their hands on the sick person's head or, unless it would be immodest or embarrassing to do so, on the affected part of the person's body, asking God to heal the distress. The prayer will be short, lasting no more than a minute or two. The prayer may be something like this: "Dear heavenly Father, Karen has come asking You to heal her of her painful leg cramps. We ask You to take the problem away. Karen, in the name of Jesus, be healed! Amen." Anointing with oil, usually by making the sign of the cross on the person's forehead, may also be done.

The whole time of ministry lasts less than five minutes, often less, and yet God honors it. Over the years I have seen many people healed in this manner. I believe it is the best way to start a person off in the ministry of healing. No personal counseling is done, no theological answers are given and, important to the apprentice, no previous experience or expertise is needed. All that is required is a belief that God can heal and a desire to be an instrument through which God can work.

Several issues arise in conjunction with altar rail ministry.

The first is the wisdom of ministering as a team and not as individuals. While God can certainly use an individual to minister healing at the altar rail, it is wiser for a team to minister. There are several reasons for this. As more people pray, added faith is present. A greater variety of spiritual gifts is present, as are wisdom and experience. While a group can go wrong in ministry, it is less likely than for an individual ministering alone. A group also offers a lessened danger of ego. When an individual prays for someone and that person is healed, he has the tendency, even though he knows better, to take the credit for the healing. Not only does this rob God of the glory due only to Him, but it puts a temptation in our paths to consider ourselves superstars. When several people minister, it is impossible to know who it was that God chose to use as the instrument for the healing to happen. And finally, it is unwise for a variety of reasons to have someone minister solo to someone of the opposite sex. Having a second team member present helps alleviate this problem.

A second issue of altar rail ministry is the spiritual phenomena that sometimes accompany a time of prayer. Someone being prayed for may be overcome by the power of the Holy Spirit in such a way that he or she falls to the floor. (This is addressed in Appendix 1.) Another phenomenon is heat—in our hands or in the place of illness in the person for whom we are praying or both. Sometimes this is a sign that God is using a particular person on the team in a special way that day. That team member might be the one to take the lead in ministry. The heat may occur in a place in the sick person's body other than where the team was devoting its attention. This may indicate additional need for prayer.

Another manifestation is a sense of tingling or shaking in our hands or in the sick person or both.

There may be, additionally, a sense—gentle or overwhelming—of the presence of God.

These phenomena do not always accompany a time of prayer. Their presence does not necessarily mean that a team member is spiritually mature, although many of the great healers, saints and mystics throughout the ages reported these phenomena. Nor does their absence necessarily mean faithlessness on the part of one praying. Sometimes they may even be counterfeits of Satan to get us distracted or puffed up with pride. Just be aware that they sometimes occur, ask God to show you what they mean and resolve that you will not be distracted by them.

A third issue that arises in altar rail ministry is the sense that God is speaking to us about the person with whom we are praying. God may be giving us discernment about the person's life. He may be giving us a word of knowledge or a word of wisdom about his situation. Such insights could either be in words, in pictures or in a general sense that in some way God is guiding our thoughts.

Often such communication from God shows either a key to the healing we are seeking, an additional problem for which we need to pray, the pathway to future spiritual growth or all three of these.

While such divine guidance has been part of the experience of the Church since her beginnings, and while old manuals on prayer and spiritual direction describe these things in detail, they are new to many.[1] As the Church rediscovers what they mean, we need to exercise caution. We want to test such purported communication to make sure it has indeed come from God. We test by making sure that such words are in conformity to Scripture (1 John 4:1). We test ourselves to see if, when we get a "word," it bears out in reality. If I believe a person has a gallbladder problem, for example, and a medical examination confirms this, I will be more confident that I can hear God speaking words of knowledge than if it is not borne out by the evidence. If it seems to be the case that God is giving us such words and that we are hearing Him correctly, we will want to make use of this information in ministry to the sick. As we do, however, we must keep a few things in mind.

First, we should use such information only after addressing the particular problem that those being prayed for first mentioned. Why? For one reason, while what they said may not actually be important, *it is important to them at this time.* They may not hear anything else we say if we are not directly focusing—at least at first—where they are focusing.

Second, they may realize that they have other, more urgent problems, but they will not trust us with them until they see how we do with a problem that is relatively safe to share.

Third, if those with whom we are praying have never heard of God's supernatural impartation of information to a person conducting ministry, or if their only experience has been negative, we could frighten them with a bold announcement that we know personal information. It could be startling for someone to hear something like this: "God just gave me a word for you, sister. He told me your problem is you won't forgive your mother." That's not ministry, that's assault! It would be much better to say: "As I was praying for you, I came to wonder if perhaps some of your need may be for reconciliation with your mother. Could that be on target?" Remember, if God prods but does not force, then we too should prod but not force. If this woman does not want to deal with the problem of unforgiveness of her mother, we must respect that. Then again, maybe we did not hear God correctly ourselves.

Yes, we should be careful in how we use words from the Lord. We do not, on the other hand, want to let our caution immobilize us. While misuse of something from God can be harmful, not to use it may block the healing someone needs.

We should not only share whatever comes to us in prayer, but we should ask the one being prayed for if anything came to his or her mind while the prayers were being offered. Always remember, the sick person is not passive in the process of healing, but an active member of the team. By encouraging him to pray and listen carefully for the voice of God, we are helping not only his physical well-being, but also his spiritual growth to further, fuller wholeness.

Please remember that various spiritual manifestations such as falling over in the power of the Holy Spirit, heat, tingling or words from the Lord can be—and historically have been—expressed in a variety of ways. We can respect but need not copy the particular cultural style of Pentecostals in order to honor the way God is working.

A healing team can also be deployed in a style of healing ministry that many call "prayer counseling." We will examine this in the next chapter.

Discussion Questions

1. What is the reason or theory for having a designated healing team?
2. Using one-word characteristics, write the minimum requirements for a healing team member.
3. Read Luke 8:40–48. Answer the questions on this passage listed in Appendix 4.

13

Ministering Healing by Prayer Counseling

Prayer counseling is a style of ministering healing different from hospital or home visitation or ministry at the altar rail. In this format, the healing team takes much more time with a person and examines his or her needs more extensively. Just as Jesus ministered to both multitudes and individuals, so the healing team operates in both settings. The setting in prayer counseling is more akin to pastoral counseling than to a service of worship. Prayer counseling is not a better way of ministering healing; it is just different. One way of ministry may be called for at one time, a different way another time.

Prayer counseling gives the team the chance to work in considerably more depth. Because of the vital interconnectedness of body, soul and spirit, the approach is whole-person in orientation. Prayer counseling makes use of all of the "sub-specialties" of healing ministry: laying on of hands, confession, inner healing, deliverance, counseling, guidance about nutrition and exercise and so on. Each of these sub-specialties has an integrity of its own. In prayer counseling they are all brought together and made use of as appropriate.

Prayer counseling may require one or several sessions to examine all aspects of a person's life, from diet, to exercise, to sleep patterns, to emotional hurts, to involvement with the occult, to spiritual strengths and weaknesses. In addition to being therapeutic, it can be preventative; presenting our lives before the Lord for improvement and scrutiny can keep any number of problems from happening. (See chapter 14, "Being and Staying Well," for an examination of those preventative measures we can take.)

As a church healing team becomes known and accepted, more and more people will seek it out for ministry. Some people come because they know something is wrong with their lives but do not know what it is. While those who can put a finger on a single problem may find it sufficient to be prayed for briefly at the altar rail, those whose problems are undefined may need a more thorough diagnostic ministry.

Some people come because they have been referred to the team by the clergy or by professional counselors. Godly pastors and trained, qualified Christian counselors are usually in such demand that they are more than happy to refer to capable lay ministers those whose problems are less severe than those needing in-depth professional care. Others come because of friends' references.

Some people come because as we (or others) minister healing to them at the altar rail, we sense that a prayer counseling format would be more effective.

Some people come because they have been prayed for at the altar rail repeatedly and nothing seems to happen. In those cases, we may sense that the causes of their dis-ease are more complex or deep-rooted than can be ministered to in a few minutes.

Finally, some people come not because anything dramatic is wrong, but just to bring their lives before the Lord to be looked at by faithful ministers. Just as having annual physical examinations is advantageous, so are sessions like this from time to time. As one's life is looked at, a number of minor things can be addressed before they become major.

It is important to conduct the prayer counseling sessions in a place where you will not be disturbed and with sufficient time for the sessions not to be rushed. It is a good rule of thumb, however, that no session last longer than an hour and a half. Any longer and the counselee gets tired and perhaps overwhelmed by having to deal with too many issues at once. Often the sessions are shorter.

Prayer counseling can be informal as a few members of the healing team meet to talk with someone desiring help. In the course of the conversation, various issues are brought up and addressed. Done in this way, prayer counseling is more like an extended version of ministry at the altar rail. With no time pressures, conversation can be relaxed and the time of prayer more extended.

There are advantages to longer soaking prayers. Sometimes the blessings of healing need to soak in gradually, just as water from a gentle rain takes time to soak into the ground. I am often surprised, when watering my garden, that even after watering for some time the soil is still dry at a small depth under the surface mud. Clearly, to reach the roots of some plants, much more watering is needed. No rule of thumb determines how long is enough, except that we often underestimate how long a time of prayer is needed.

If the person desiring ministry is known to the team, the initial time of light conversation before ministry begins can be brief. Fewer questions need to be asked. The sessions could take place in the person's home. If the person desiring ministry is not known to the team, however, other dynamics come into play.

First, the initial time of light conversation needs to be somewhat longer so the counselee can relax and become comfortable with the team members. This is important so trust can be established. As the team members get to know the counselee, they begin to understand his or her inner dynamics. Counselees sometimes have difficulty expressing their inner feelings or are honestly unaware of them. By getting to know the people we are counseling, we can help them express what they are feeling and become aware of what is going on inside.

Second, more attention needs to be given initially to discovering the various roots of the counselee's problems. The diagnostic checklist in Appendix 2 may prove helpful here. This checklist is consciously modeled on the intake interview that a physician does in a complete history and physical, only it goes further. The purpose is to get, as thoroughly as possible, a look at the life of the person we are trying to help.

It could be that only a few issues stand out as needing attention. In that case, ministry can be accomplished in one or two sessions and with the two or three people from the team who are present.

If it looks as though several problems will need addressing, however, a more thorough approach is called for. One person from the team should be assigned as "case manager." This term is borrowed from social work. It refers to the person who, in the multiplicity of various helping persons, makes sure that the person being helped gets the assistance needed in a well-integrated fashion and does not feel chopped up among various specialists. The case manager takes notes on what is done in each session and makes sure that if additional assistance is needed, such persons are brought on board. The case manager also makes sure that all the aspects of ministry are well-coordinated. With many ministering according to their specialties in the ministry of healing, this is quite important.

In these cases, the team may need to be augmented by other individuals from the team or even by individuals who are not part of your church's healing team. The fact is, no one minister of healing can adequately handle the whole variety of issues a seriously hurting person has. As the apostle Paul points out (1 Corinthians 12:4), there are a variety of gifts. While God occasionally uses an individual in gifts in which he or she seldom ministers, God normally makes use of several individuals ministering together, each with his or her own contribution to the healing process.

Third, it is a good idea to conduct a prayer counseling session with a person not known to the team in the church and not in a private home.

Before ministry begins, it is important to determine if the person we are counseling actually wants to be healed. Jesus asked this of the man at the pool of Bethesda (John 5:6). If someone does not want to be healed, you are wasting your time and his. Some people so enjoy being ministered to that they refuse to be healed. They tenaciously cling to their problems so that others will keep ministering to them. We can actually harm them by reinforcing and rewarding their neuroses if we play along! This is not to say that they do not have a problem. They obviously do. But their need is for someone to go to the root of the real problem, not the one they present to us. Their need may be for someone to "tough love" them into responsible behavior, not to affirm their dead-end expressions of self-pity or victimization. If you are not experienced enough in prayer counseling to discern this, or if you are but the counselees are not willing to let you expose their real problems, no progress can occur.

We also need to determine before ministry begins whether or not the counselees will do their homework. The ministry of prayer counseling involves not only the cooperation of those being counseled but their active participation as well. It is *their* lives that are in need. We cannot take what is there and overlay wholeness on top. They need renewing from within, which cannot happen without their active participation. At the end of each session, the team should assign the counselee some homework. At the next session, begin by asking how the homework assignment went. If little or nothing was done, stop the session immediately and tell him or her that you cannot resume until the homework assignment is completed.

It may sound cruel to break off ministry if the person refuses to let us work on a deeper problem. But remember, our purpose is to bring people into wholeness. Sometimes we may be so eager to be active in ministry that we care more for the good feeling of ministering than we do for the welfare of the other person. It may be that we have to be strict for them to take the process seriously. If they do not, others who are serious about healing need our time.

Prayer, of course, is an essential component of prayer counseling. Far from being a mere formality—like those obligatory prayers offered at certain public gatherings—prayer is at the heart of what we are about. The team should pray together before the counselee arrives. Each session should begin with prayer, inviting the counselee to pray as well. We should ask God to guide, direct and protect the session, and to pour His love and grace upon the counselee and His wisdom and power upon the members of the team.

The team should not only encourage the counselee to pray as team members pray at various points in the counseling session, but instruct the counselee how to do it if he or she is not able to do so. Not only are we prayer partners with those we are trying to help; we are also spiritual coaches. The point is not to make them dependent on us, but rather to present them mature in Christ (Colossians 1:28). Our desire is not only to be agents of God's healing, but also instructors in spiritual growth.

After praying for the counselee for a while, we can stop to ask if he or she feels any different. This is true in those cases where the problem is one of an outward physical condition. While we cannot tell short of a blood test whether or not God has healed a problem with cholesterol, we can tell immediately if there is any change in one's shoulder pain or leg mobility, for example.

This is also true in cases where the problem is emotional or spiritual. While change in these areas often comes gradually, there are times when the breakthrough is rapid. Suddenly the counselee becomes aware that a burden has been lifted or a fear has left.

When a healing has indeed taken place, we should stop to praise and thank God. God did something, and realizing this causes faith to grow. It will be easier to believe Him for the other needed healings to take place. Or, if a partial healing has occurred, we thank God for what He has done and ask Him to complete His work.

Let me give you an example of how a series of prayer counseling sessions might take place with a person whose problems are complex in nature. For this example (based on real life), I will call the case manager Doris, her church Morningside United Methodist Church and the person needing ministry Andrea Johnston.

Andrea was referred to Morningside Church by a friend who knew that the Lord was doing good things there. Andrea's request for ministry was passed on by the church secretary to the head of the healing team, who passed it in turn on to Doris, one of the team members. Doris called Andrea. They chatted on the telephone for several minutes so Doris could sense if Andrea was serious about being helped, determine whether Andrea's problems were within the range of what the healing team could handle (or if a referral to a Christian counselor was necessary) and establish the beginning of a relationship. A time for the first appointment was set.

At the first session, Doris, Andrea and Michael Braddock, another member of the team, spent several minutes getting to know each other. After a time of prayer, Doris explained the process of healing through prayer counseling. Doris then asked Andrea to repeat the reasons why she was seeking ministry. Andrea said there was not anything in particular that stood out; she just didn't feel good.

As Doris went through the diagnostic checklist (again, Appendix 2), several problem areas became apparent. Andrea's problems were: (1) stomach aches; (2) difficulty in praying (when she tried to pray, which wasn't that often); (3) the matter of having stolen a few things at work; (4) fear that her father would die and that she would be left all alone; and (5) an admission that she had been to several séances.

Doris first got Andrea's promise that she would get a complete physical and tell her physician of the stomach complaints. Doris did not know if the stomach problem might be reflux, ulcers, cancer or something else. She told Andrea that sometimes a physical problem can come from a variety of sources. "It might come from a disease, from trauma due to a fall or from the body just breaking down," she said. "It might be the result of emotional or spiritual distress. In any case, whatever the cause or causes, the problem needs to be addressed."

Michael pointed out that God could heal the problem miraculously, through medicine or through the process of prayer counseling. They stopped at this point to pray for healing, and suggested that until the problem ceased, it might be wise to see what medicine or diet modification would be useful in alleviating the symptoms.

Then Doris addressed the matter of stealing. She told Andrea that while God is loving and forgiving, we must turn from our sins, make restitution for what we have done wrong and reaffirm our desire to obey Jesus as Lord over our lives. She tried to help Andrea understand that it is not only individual acts that concern God, but the whole orientation of our lives. The ultimate question is not "Did I do a particular thing wrong?" but "Am I actively trying to make Jesus Lord over my life?" Doris said that it would be important for Andrea to conduct a thorough examination of her life in accordance with the revealed will of God in Scripture. She could do that with a layperson in an informal manner, or with a minister or priest as a formal confession. In either case, it needed to be done. As Doris was not a member of the clergy, nor did she or Michael feel gifted in helping another person to examine her life and repent of her sins, she said she would be happy to arrange for Andrea to see either a pastor or a person on the healing team who was gifted in these matters.

Andrea admitted that this would probably be a good idea, yet questioned what relevancy it had to her stomach difficulties. Doris took some time to explain the interconnectedness of body, soul and spirit. She told Andrea how her stomach problem could have come from any number of sources—from food poisoning, guilt about having stolen, her fear of losing her father, a demonic attack from her opening herself up to evil spirits at a séance or from any number of other sources. Michael told Andrea that while we do not always know what the cause of a problem is, the thoroughness of prayer counseling often gets to the roots.

Time for the first session was up. While Doris, Michael and Andrea would have liked to continue, they had been at it for almost an hour and a half. Andrea had homework to do: She had to get her complete physical, she needed to make thorough confession of her sins and she needed to do the Scripture reading Doris had assigned her. It was enough to keep her busy for two weeks. Doris and Michael prayed again for Andrea's stomach troubles to be healed and for God to assist her in doing her homework. They made an appointment to meet again. As they were leaving, Michael reminded Andrea that even if the stomach problems were to go away in the meantime, she should still keep their next appointment for two reasons: first, God had a wonderful supply of blessings to give Andrea, and second, she could grow further in the knowledge that Jesus was her Lord. The urgency of these two things should not be short-circuited in case the problem that brought Andrea to prayer counseling was removed.

Two weeks later, Andrea came back. Doris first asked her if she had gone to the doctor. Andrea replied that her doctor was heavily booked up but that she had made an appointment with her for later that week. Andrea volunteered that she had met with Jim Nagle, the associate pastor of Morningside Church. She and Pastor Jim had examined a number of areas in her life that needed change and she said that they would be examining them further to see how she could do just that. Doris said she would need to be in touch with Pastor Jim, not to find out specific details, but so that the people working to help Andrea would be working in harmony. Andrea agreed to write a one-sentence note authorizing Doris, Michael and Pastor Nagle to share necessary information.

In the two weeks between appointments, Doris had been praying for wisdom as to what issue in Andrea's life to tackle next. Was it Andrea's fear of being left alone? If it was fear, was the fear emotional in origin, was it a demon of fear, or both? If both, which should be addressed first? If fear was not the issue to be addressed next, was it Andrea's involvement with the occult? Doris knew that there is no automatic, textbook answer to the question of the order in which ministry should be done. Waiting for a word from God was crucial. Doris knew, further, that if inner healing was next, she would need to pray to discern who on the team gifted in inner healing would be the right one to minister to Andrea. She also knew that if deliverance prayer was to happen next, she would want to know who should supplement her own gift in that area.

Doris came away from her time of waiting for the Lord's answer with some sense of God's direction, but nothing clear-cut. This used to trouble Doris, but over three years of ministering healing she had come to believe that while sometimes one proceeds with clear, unmistakable guidance from the Lord, at other times one proceeds on the basis of an educated guess. Her pride no longer made her embarrassed if she had to admit a different tack was needed because the one she was on was not getting results. She smiled, realizing it was exactly the way her cousin Ed, a physician, worked.

Just as Doris was about to start the second session, Andrea said, "Can we talk about the best way for me to make amends for the things I stole from work?" Doris knew that sometimes the minister of healing has to set the agenda but at other times the person to whom we are ministering directs it. This seemed to be one of those times.

Talking and praying through the issue of restitution took so much time that there was little time left for anything else. Doris felt that to begin to work now on something else would be unwise as it would be rushed or cut short. She asked Andrea how she was doing on her Scripture reading. Andrea admitted she had put it off for no good reason. Doris laughingly scolded Andrea, telling her that Scripture study was as important as taking the pills the doctor gives us. Andrea agreed to do better. Doris told Andrea that they would be working on issues raised by her involvement in the occult at the next session.

"Oh, I wasn't in the occult," said Andrea. "I'm not into any of that Satan stuff I've been seeing on TV."

Doris felt this was not the time to point out that there are many seemingly harmless things that are occultish and against God. Instead she asked Andrea to read a small introductory book on spiritual warfare so that Andrea would know what the next session would be about. She agreed. An appointment for two weeks later was made.

Just as Andrea was going through the doorway, Doris yelled out, "Oh, I almost forgot! How's your stomach?"

"Good!" Andrea replied. "Haven't had a problem in over a week."

With a smile on her face, Doris asked, "Then why did you come back?"

"Because," Andrea replied thoughtfully, "I see how important getting everything in my life in order is. I want it for God and I want it for me. I want to get the garbage out and the good stuff in. And I know you care about me."

Andrea called Doris four days later to tell her there was some good news and some bad news. The good news was that her efforts at restitution went well. Her boss was amazed that she went to him, confessed what she had done and laid a check covering what was stolen on the table between them.

He was so amazed he said he would not prosecute her for theft, something that Andrea was prepared for even though she was praying hard and often that it would not happen. The bad news was that her doctor found she had a moderate case of esophageal reflux but that it could be controlled with diet modification and could be alleviated with medication if it got too bad.

Doris rejoiced with Andrea. She did not remind her of her other homework, hoping that the good feeling Andrea had over making restitution would be all the encouragement she needed.

Ten days later the three of them met again. As always, they spent a few minutes chatting about "life," began with prayer and discussed how things had been going since the last visit. Andrea had been doing her Bible studies and had even gone with a girlfriend to a midweek prayer meeting at a charismatic Presbyterian church. But no, she had not read the book on spiritual warfare.

"Please don't take this as rejection, Andrea," Doris said. "But I think it's important that you have a basic understanding of the spiritual world—of good and evil spirits and how these things work—before we work on your deliverance. We can reschedule the appointment for a week from now if that's O.K."

Andrea understood and thanked Doris for being "professional."

"We don't like to use the word *professional* in terms of ministry," Doris replied. "But I know what you mean."

A week later they met again. Andrea had read the book. There were parts of it she did not understand, and a few places where she thought the author was being unnecessarily narrow. The most important thing she derived from the book, however, was that there is a spiritual battle going on and she had innocently opened herself up for possible harm.

Doris told Andrea that sometimes she discerned the presence of the demonic. Andrea now knew enough to know what those words meant and was concerned. "No," Doris responded, "I don't sense anything with you. That doesn't mean there isn't anything to deal with, however. No one's discernment is one hundred percent accurate. But not to worry, God is stronger than any evil power."

Michael first led Andrea in a prayer of renunciation of Satan and all his works. (See Appendix 5.) Then he asked Andrea if she had ever accepted Jesus as her Savior and Lord. Andrea replied that she remembered doing that when she was confirmed in the Episcopal Church as a teenager. When Doris asked if she had understood what her vows meant and if she was genuine in her commitment, Andrea replied, "Yes, very much so. I guess I drifted away from it over the years, but at the time our priest explained thoroughly why we need a Savior and how Jesus is Savior and Lord." Doris led Andrea in a prayer of rededication. (See an example in Appendix 5.)

Then Doris and Michael asked the Holy Spirit to fill spots made empty by any departing evil spirits. (See what Jesus said about this in Matthew 12:43–45.)

When that was over Andrea asked, "Is that it?" Doris didn't know what Andrea meant so Andrea explained, "I was expecting shouting and screaming on your part and me speaking with a deep bass voice and all that!"

"Oh, no!" Doris hastened to reply. "Don't believe everything you see in those movies and TV shows. Some of it is exaggerated, and even the parts that are true occur in only a small percentage of the cases. Often when I pray for deliverance, nothing noticeable happens. But people comment that heaviness seems to lift from their spirits and they find prayer, worship and Bible reading to be much easier. Sometimes troublesome thoughts go away, too. Other times there are a few outward manifestations of the demonic, like twitching or jerking of the person's body as I command the evil spirits to leave. I never raise my voice because, for one thing, the demons aren't deaf; for another, they respond to the authority God grants believers; and third, why scare people unnecessarily? Sometimes when I pray there are probably no evil spirits present. What I'm doing, then, is saying, in effect, 'I don't know if you're there, but if you are, get lost in Jesus' name.'" They both laughed.

After this, Doris gave Andrea some help on how to win in her battle over temptation. Doris instructed Andrea what things are demonic, occultic and New Age, and, therefore, forbidden by God and harmful to us. Her homework assignment for Andrea was basic Christian discipleship teaching on spiritual growth, prayer, worship and Scripture study. They agreed to meet three weeks later.

After the usual pleasantries, now growing a bit longer as the three had grown in their friendship, was the time of prayer. For the first time, and quite spontaneously, Andrea offered a brief prayer. She was pleased at that, yet admitted it lacked the formal structure of Doris' more experienced words. Doris and Michael assured Andrea that God looked first on the heart and last on the form.

Doris did two things she had not done before. First, she asked Andrea if she was worshiping regularly on Sunday. Andrea gave Doris a look as if wondering if the price of her healing was to join Morningside Church! Doris understood immediately and told Andrea that while of course they would welcome her with open arms at Morningside Church, she did not have to attend there as long as she was worshiping in a place that would nurture her newly rediscovered Christian discipleship. Andrea said that because of her work schedule, Sunday was impossible, but that she had not missed a Wednesday night prayer meeting at the Presbyterian church in two months.

Second, Doris asked if she could present some of the details of what had been happening during the sessions of prayer counseling to her healing team meeting. "From time to time we each need to make a presentation to the group of the work we are doing. This helps us all learn and it particularly benefits the person making the presentation, because anything we may be doing wrong as we minister is examined and corrected."

Andrea was a bit concerned. "You won't . . . I'm not sure what I mean; but you won't. . . ."

"Blab all your secrets?" Doris offered. "No, of course not. Remember the word *professional* you used last session? While you'll remember I don't like the word, you could say that we are certainly as discreet as any professional counselor or physician. And if there are parts of what we've been discussing that you don't want shared, please tell me, and I'll work around those."

"No, I trust you, Doris. You have my permission to discuss my situation with your colleagues."

Michael asked Andrea about her fears of abandonment and of losing her father. "The fears are still there," Andrea responded. Michael explained that sometimes fears—or other unwanted emotions—disappear at a session of deliverance. "Other times they don't. This is either because the need for deliverance is much deeper—which I don't sense here—or else the fears were caused by something other than evil spirits. My sense is that what's needed here is inner healing." They took several minutes to explain what that was.

"We're not particularly gifted in that area," Michael explained. "We do have someone on our healing team named Marcy Bates who is not only gifted in inner healing but seems to have her best results in matters dealing with women and their fathers. I'd like to bring her into our work, if you don't mind."

"Please do, but on one condition," Andrea responded. "I want you two present when these 'inner healing' things occur."

Doris laughed. "Don't worry. Inner healing doesn't bite and you're not made to look foolish. It *would* make it easier if we were there, because our desire is not only to be your friend and do our part in helping you toward wholeness, but remember, I'm the one who coordinates the efforts of the others who are helping you. By being there, we could be plugged in firsthand. But you need to know that we will be saying and doing very little except praying and making occasional observations. Marcy will be doing more of the direct ministry."

Andrea felt comfortable with that, although she was surprised to learn that the ministry of inner healing usually takes much longer than that of confession or deliverance. In the case of Andrea Johnston, it did take longer. In fact, Andrea, Michael, Doris and Marcy worked at it for a total of eleven sessions.[1] They prayed for God's wisdom and guidance prior to the first session, and God did not let them down.

In the middle of the first session, Marcy felt she had gotten a word of knowledge that Andrea had been left behind somewhere and that was the—or at least a—source of her fear of abandonment. Although Andrea did not recollect an incident, her father did. When she was a little girl, they had gone to the mall together and she had disobeyed him by wandering off. They wondered out loud together if that was why she was so fearful whenever her dad, a salesman, went away on a business trip. Andrea marveled at how much a blessing the gifts of the Holy Spirit are to God's people.

At each session of inner healing they asked Jesus to remove Andrea's fears about being abandoned. They suggested that several times during the day she picture in her mind's eye Jesus standing next to her. Once Andrea, with childlike giggles, shared how funny she thought it was that Jesus went shopping with her to Kmart. "He seemed to enjoy it!" she added.

In addition to ministering inner healing, Doris, Michael and Marcy made sure that Andrea was growing spiritually. They checked in occasionally with Pastor Jim Nagle to see how Andrea was doing in matters of repentance. Whenever it seemed that Andrea was becoming a passive recipient of their ministry, they made her take responsibility not only for her healing, but for her growth in Christ as well.

They showed her how the various parts of healing inter-connect, not just in theory, but in real life, and not just at the beginning of ministry, but at all times. This careful instruction bore fruit in the sixth session of inner healing when Andrea suddenly realized she had never forgiven her father for losing track of her at the mall.

"You know, I love my father, but I haven't forgiven him for that. And I used to tell him he was selfish for going on his business trips without taking me."

Neither Doris, Michael nor Marcy sensed any animosity on the part of Andrea toward her father. In fact, they sensed much love. But they realized that they could not know every-thing. Maybe Andrea still harbored resentment. Besides, thought Michael, Andrea's realization of unforgiveness did not seem to be a neurotic sense of false guilt.

"O.K., here's what I suggest," responded Marcy. "You're learning how to pray out loud and informally. Let's have a prayer in which you ask God to forgive you for whatever resentment you harbored or still harbor against your father." After this was done, they talked about whether it was neces-sary for Andrea to ask her father's forgiveness for what she did as a child.

The outcome of the sessions of inner healing was that Andrea Johnston was set free. Her reflux still kicks up from time to time, usually after a big dinner. But she is a new per-son in several ways. She has grown much closer to the Lord and she is more whole emotionally and spiritually. At last report, Andrea was taking the healing ministry training course at Morningside United Methodist Church so she could find out how God could use her in ministry to others.

The expression of the healing ministry called prayer coun-seling can take place in any church in which there are godly people who take it seriously and believe God can use them in service to others. While not as exciting, perhaps, as the sudden dramatic healings that take place at a healing service, it is an opportunity to apply the riches of Christ's transforming power to people in ways that are thorough, deep and lasting.

Discussion Questions

1. What kinds of situations do you perceive as appropriate for prayer counseling, rather than one of the other forms of ministry?
2. Read the Diagnostic Checklist in Appendix 2. Ask yourself the questions and honestly record the answers. Record any conclusions about your own wholeness.
3. What are the essential ingredients of prayer counseling?
4. In ministering to an individual, list the advantages and disadvantages of team ministry.

14

Being and Staying Well
Mary Grace Pearson, D.O.

Being well is more than being healed, and health is more than not being sick. Often we settle for the absence of sickness rather than the abundant life Jesus came to bring us (John 10:10). In this chapter we will discuss how to be well and how to seek the abundant life—physical, emotional and spiritual—that Jesus promised us.

Physical

We often shrug off exercise and diet as the field of health nuts. Nonetheless, in pursuing health we need to examine these issues carefully. Most people who attempt to diet or exercise their bodies into shape fail, and they fail for the same reasons. Because of their failures, they dismiss these disciplines of life as impossible. Why do people fail?

1. Unrealistic goals. Many people expect to lose thirty pounds in one month. Or they imagine themselves exercising their bodies into figures that sixteen-year-olds would be proud of—in a few weeks! This is why fad diets and paid weight loss plans are popular and ultimately fail.

2. Unrealistic plans. Some of us make dramatic resolutions about exercising an hour every day. We plan on waking up at 5 A.M., going for a three-mile jog, lifting weights and dancing through an exercise video as soon as we get home from work. Many will stop after the first bout of muscle aches and pains, but most stop after they are thrown off their carefully planned schedule one too many times after getting home late from work or staying up late with a sick child. An unrealistic plan ultimately dooms us to failure.

3. Lack of persistence. We get bored. We get tired. We get discouraged at our lack of results. And we realize that ultimately we are more comfortable watching baseball than playing it. We binge or forget to exercise, then abuse ourselves instead of saying, "Whoops, guess I'll try harder next time."

So how can we overcome our inclinations to overeat and underexercise?

Any change we make in our lives must be based in the Lord. "Unless the Lord builds the house, those who build it labor in vain" (Psalm 127:1). We need to repent of any gluttony or neglect of the temple in which we dwell (1 Corinthians 6:19). We need to ask God's direction in our lives, especially regarding our attitudes toward food, wellness and our own bodies. We need to ask God's help in establishing realistic goals and plans.

Now let me be clear. Realistic goals are important. Self-control is a fruit of the Holy Spirit (Galatians 5:23). Looking like a model is not. Many Christians, particularly young women, get themselves into trouble at this point. In fact, the Bible urges women in particular not to focus on outward beauty but on developing a godly character (1 Peter 3:3–4). So how do we establish realistic goals?

Diet

Food intake should be determined by our needs, not just our wants. An eighty-year-old-woman and an eighteen-year-old man will have different food requirements. Of benefit to everyone is a diet high in fruits, vegetables and complex carbohydrates and adequate water. It is generally recommended that most people maintain a low-fat diet (a caloric intake of less than thirty percent fat). Although we do need some fat in our diet, most of us need less than one tablespoon a day! There is another benefit of a low-fat diet. Since fat is calorie-dense, fat makes you fat and low-fat foods do not! Foods that are low in fat are breads, pastas, fish, vegetables and fruits. Butter, margarine, fatty meats (especially red meat), fried foods and dairy products (except skim milk or foods made from skim milk) are high in fat.

There is some evidence that a diet with between 5–6 servings of fruits and vegetables a day protects against cancer. There is much evidence that a low-fat diet helps prevent heart disease. A healthy diet includes a wide variety of fresh fruits, vegetables, complex carbohydrates (bread, pasta, cereal), low-fat dairy products, lean meat and fish. These should make up *at least seventy percent* of all the calories in your diet, preferably 85%. One of the many little books in the supermarkets can tell you the fat and calorie content of each food.

Some foods must be used cautiously at all times. These are caffeine, alcohol and salt. Note that I did not say *should not be used*, merely *used cautiously*. Let me explain.

Caffeine is a stimulant chemical found primarily in coffee, colas, tea and chocolate. It heightens awareness and alertness (thus its popularity with students, long-distance drivers and workers on the night shift). Unfortunately, caffeine can contribute to restlessness, insomnia, rapid heartbeat and irritability. In some people it can cause diarrhea, aggravate irritable bowel syndrome, even set off a migraine headache. There is also some evidence that women who consume coffee prior to and during their pregnancies have a higher rate of miscarriage.

In general, caffeine for most people in small amounts (less than four cups of coffee per day) is harmless. Caffeine is generally a problem only when it is consumed in excess. If you have any symptoms of irritability, restlessness, insomnia, anxiety or rapid heartbeat, however, consider stopping all your caffeine intake.

Alcohol is a substance with a long history of medicinal use and social abuse. Timothy was advised by none other than the apostle Paul to take a little wine to help his stomach (1 Timothy 5:23). Some recent evidence, in fact, indicates that wine, used moderately, can help prevent heart disease. (Moderate means one or two drinks of four ounces each.) Unfortunately, some people are alcoholics and cannot use alcohol in moderation. For them alcohol becomes an addictive substance destroying liver, heart, brain—even life itself. Those who suffer from alcoholism live most productively when they abstain from alcohol use altogether. Even people who are not alcoholics can be sensitive to its side effects, including fatigue, impaired judgment, flushing and confusion. These people may need to avoid alcohol, too, not because of an addiction but because of their sensitivity to it.

Alcohol, even white wine, is high in calories and needs to be calculated into your diet. No one should use alcohol before driving, hunting or operating machinery. We need only to read the newspapers to see how these can be tragic combinations.

Salt is a flavoring as well as a preservative. When Jesus referred to us as the salt of the earth (Matthew 5:13), He compared us to something that improves the flavor of the world and helps keep it from rotting. In ancient and recent times, salt was used as a preservative—for example, salt cod and salt pork. Salt enhances other flavors, too, as well as provides flavor of its own. Anyone who has tried unsalted tortilla chips knows they are just not as tasty!

Unfortunately, salt has the effect of elevating our blood pressures and making us retain fluid. This is more significant for some people than for others. For someone who has a normal blood pressure and is in good general health, the occasional use of salt is probably not harmful. Anyone with fluid retention problems or heart disease, on the other hand, should probably avoid salt as much as possible. Individuals of African ancestry often have a superior salt-conserving mechanism, which makes them more susceptible to the effects of salt and more prone to elevated blood pressure and subsequent heart disease.

As with all things, our diets should be moderate. Believe it or not, the reason many people fail in their diets is that the diets are too strict. People give up on the diet because they feel "it's not worth it," or because when they are over at Aunt Tilly's house they will hurt Aunt Tilly's feelings if they don't have a slice of her double chocolate torte. Have a piece! (Have a *small* piece.) Just don't go home the next day and make some more! Have whatever you like—in small amounts. Don't cheat every day. When you fail on your diet, don't give up. Start again.

Exercise

While all of us would like to have the firm body of a professional athlete, most of us do not have eight spare hours a day to exercise. The following is not meant as a guide to start Olympic training, then; it is meant as a guide to keep you fit within the dictates of your schedule. "Not *my* schedule," you might be thinking. Yes, *your* schedule.

First, commit your course to the Lord. Ask Him for help in being physically fit. Ask Him to show you where in your schedule you can find the time to exercise.

Second, look for the "wasted" time in your schedule. What do you do during commercials? Is there time while you are on hold on the telephone? While you wait for someone to call? While you wait for the washing machine at the laundromat? While you wait in airports? Look for these time slots, whether they are minutes or hours. Doing some sit-ups and pushups or stretching exercises during commercials will keep you fit better than trotting out to the kitchen for another bag of Doritos. Stretching or doing isometric exercises will help tone you even during those brief times. Walking in the airport will help you stay limber as you await your flight. **Third,** find out what kind of exercise you like to do. (It is with great difficulty that I have persuaded Mark that listening to the Red Sox does not constitute exercise!) We like to walk. When that is not feasible in our New England climate, we go to the local mall to walk. Some people have a pool available to them at or near work. Others like to play racquetball or tennis on their lunch hour.

The single best thing to remember when converting from couch potatohood is that *something* is better than nothing. There are indications that even a slow-paced stroll twice a week improves fitness in sedentary individuals. So figure out what you can do—and *do it* !

Another important component of physical well-being is rest. This is probably the single-most neglected aspect of well-being in America. It is a rare week that someone does not come into my office with fatigue, wondering why they cannot balance a forty-hour work week, a family and an aggressive social life, all on four to five hours of sleep per night! Many people are proud of how little sleep they can get by on. When I was a medical resident, we looked admiringly at the person who needed the least sleep: "He only needs four hours a night. Think of all that extra time he has!"

Scripture, in contrast, says, "It is in vain that you rise up early and go late to rest, eating the bread of anxious toil; for he gives to his beloved sleep" (Psalm 127:2). We try to maximize the quality of our lives by doing more. Yet all we accomplish is ill health, snoozing during our devotions and depending on caffeine to keep us going.

I am not proposing to set up sleep as the new idol. Any parent who has stayed up with a sick child knows there are times when sleep must be sacrificed. I am talking about maintaining a balance in one's life. What are some sensible guidelines?

The average person needs between seven and nine hours of sleep per night. Only you can determine what makes you feel rested the next morning when you get up. You should plan to get that amount of sleep at night. A lack of sleep makes us irritable, less productive and less able to listen to God in our quiet times. To plan to get an adequate amount of sleep requires discipline. Yes, you must stop working earlier or turn off the TV earlier in the evening. You may have to settle for a less than perfectly clean house. You may have to give up an extra meeting or night out each week. It demands self-control and a decision that God will be in control of your schedule.

Secondly, you should plan one day of rest per week. A few years ago Mark and I started taking one "play day" together a week. Ideally for us this includes sleeping late, time for prayer, some enjoyable exercise (usually a walk) and some form of play. We take turns choosing what that play is; it can be anything from hiking to attending a performance of the Nutcracker ballet. The incentive to do this for workaholics: We find that our productivity increases immensely in the remaining six days. It helps open up lines of communication between us, helps alleviate anxiety and helps us maintain a clearer focus on our priorities.

Everyone's day off will be different. Our friends David and Audrey, who run a busy oceanarium in Bar Harbor, Maine, often turn on their answering machine and retreat to a quiet room in their house facing the ocean, a room well supplied with books and Bibles. They feel drained after the demands of their work and find it refreshing to spend their time quietly.

Jesus said, "The sabbath was made for man" (Mark 2:27), because He knew we need it! It is especially important for families with children to make this effort, because children need rest, too. There have been many articles about how many middle-, upper-middle and upper-class children are pushed, pushed, pushed to succeed, increasing their stress. The happiest times in my childhood were the family vacations, days stolen to hunt and fish with my father and lunches with my mom. Perhaps we need rest to rediscover rest.

Emotional

We all have emotional needs, though sometimes we ignore them. This area, like every area in our lives, needs to be balanced. Some people become obsessed with their emotional needs and histories, feeding into the victimology that troubles our society. The purpose of our examining our emotional needs and histories is not to become self-centered but to become God-centered.

Emotionally we all have a history. Some of us have had a pleasant childhood, others a difficult one. All of us have come into some sorrow or loss and dealt with it in some way, either well or poorly. We have all had emotional models around us whom to some degree we have emulated. Why is it important for us to be aware of these things? Because who we have been and how our experiences have shaped us will determine our responses in the future.

If we have grown up in a family where food is considered a source of comfort, we may be prone to overeat. If we have been part of a dysfunctional family system, we may use our Christianity as a happy gloss to cover our deepest hurts, and never allow God or our church family to help us heal or cope with our other problems. We may not know how to confront other people lovingly and appropriately, and may go to the extreme of either highly emotional confrontations over trivial issues or to caving in to other people's demands. It is not within the scope of this chapter to discuss the dynamics of family life or how to deal with emotional trauma in our past. (In the bibliography you will find several books on these issues.) I simply want to point out that in order to have emotional health, it is critical to evaluate the health of our roots and how they affect our behavior now.

Our emotional well-being is also based in the relationships we sustain. While some of these relationships are entered into volitionally (for instance, marriage or friendship), others are mandated by circumstance. You cannot, for instance, choose your parents or your customers. Although, again, the complexity of human relationships is beyond the scope of this chapter, I would like to touch on a few aspects of human relationships that are critical to emotional health.

Communication

While we all communicate differently because of our personalities,[1] there are several common elements to good communication.

Honesty is an important element. Good communication can never be based on anything but truth. While we all want to say the most comfortable thing, that is seldom helpful and often gets us into hot water later on.

With honesty must come tact. Tact is nothing more than thinking for a moment before speaking—thinking about how we would like information to be communicated to *us*. While there are some truths that are so painful that no matter how you tell someone, he or she will be hurt (for instance, telling someone she has cancer), the vast majority of information can be communicated in such a way as to affirm the person involved and honestly communicate the information necessary.

Listening is perhaps the most important aspect of communication. We all find it difficult to listen carefully to another person for any length of time. But it is important to listen, and confirm as much with positive physical gestures such as nods and eye contact (especially when dealing with an emotionally charged issue), and by occasionally repeating and rephrasing what the other person has said: "What I hear you saying is. . . ." This helps us to avoid misunderstanding what the other person is saying.

Attitude

It has always amazed me that people respond so differently to illness. One patient will be difficult, withdrawn or demanding, focused on the unfairness of the situation. Another person with an identical ailment will be cheerful, joking, grateful to God for all He has done. "It's a hard thing," they might say, "but I've had a good life, and that's more than a lot of people." This is not to say that these people do not have down times or that they do not appropriately express pain or sorrow. They simply have the "gratitude attitude." Not surprisingly, they do better overall in recovery. If we do not have this attitude naturally or have not had it instilled in us during childhood, what can we do to cultivate it?

One thing I have had to learn—being a problem-solver by nature and vocation who tends to focus immediately on problems in any given situation—is to look for the positive aspects. I need to be intentional about expressing thanks to God *before* my petitions to God. And I need to remember to thank other people for what they do for me. It does not mean I overlook problems or pretend they are going away on their own. It simply means I am committed to looking at God's goodness and faithfulness as well as my problems. Even when it seems mechanical, I find that I begin to internalize my external positive actions and begin to *feel* more grateful.

Responsibility

Emotional health is developed and protected by an appropriate sense of responsibility. Human beings tend to make one of two errors: taking responsibility for things they should not, or not taking the responsibility that is appropriate.

Part of the normal developmental process is developing appropriate boundaries between ourselves and others. We begin to understand as small children that we are different from Mommy and Daddy. That is why two-year-olds focus on "I want do it myself, Mommy" or on the dreaded *no* word. It is important for these little tykes to learn the *no* word, as frustrating as that is. Some adults have never really learned to say no and end up burned out and out of control because they cannot refuse engagements, responsibility or temptation. Illness of all sorts is more likely when burnout has pre-pared the way. The word *no* helps us to avoid responsibility that is not ours, and to form appropriate boundaries with other people.

I must admit my frustration, on the other hand, with the three-pack-a-day smoker who curses God when he is diag-nosed with lung cancer, or the fourteen-year-old girl who complains about her pregnancy with "Why did this happen to me?" How we choose to behave *does* affect our lives. We have a legitimate responsibility to take care of our bodies, minds and souls that only we can fulfill. Denying this respon-sibility can only cause pain for ourselves and others. It also keeps us from becoming emotionally mature.

Learning an appropriate responsibility for our own actions, and allowing others to take responsibility for their own actions, is critical to our emotional health. We also need to allow God sovereignty in situations that lie outside of our control. Much of our stress comes when we do not let God take charge of situations we cannot control anyway. When we find ourselves anxious and worried about things we can-not alter, we must remember the formula found in Philippi-ans: "Have no anxiety about anything, but in everything by prayer and supplication with thanksgiving let your requests be made known to God. And the peace of God, which passes all understanding, will keep your hearts and your minds in Christ Jesus" (Philippians 4:6–7). Look at this passage closely. Often when we are filled with anxiety, we try to deny that the thing we fear will come upon us; or we try to ignore the anxiety; or we feel guilty for being worried. Instead, the scrip-tural pattern is to offer all our troubles to God and to remem-ber to give thanks.

Why is giving thanks so important? First of all, God's Word commands it. Second, God deserves it. Third, it takes our minds off the negative and puts us into a more positive frame of mind. Fourth, it reminds us that God has done great things in the past and that He can do them again.

It is important that we do not deny the reality of our problems, but instead focus on God's power to solve them.

Spiritual

Spiritual health can be found only when we are in a right relationship with God. Sin is one of the major blocks to wellness (see chapter 5). Sin can be overcome only by:

1. Recognition of the sin. We all wear cultural blinders that make us perceive things differently than God does. Until perhaps twenty years ago, for instance, a woman in India would be burned to death when her husband's body was cremated. Most of us see that as the destruction of human life and deplore the callousness that allows or mandates such a custom. But as Americans we have become deadened to the aborting of almost two million fetuses each year. We do not get upset about divorce because it is a fact of life. We turn a blind eye when people in our churches have sex outside of heterosexual marriage. We ignore the plight of the poor and dismiss cheating on our income tax as a business ploy. Whatever our particular bias, we ignore our own sins and the sins of others.

2. Confession of sin. To recognize sin is not enough. God wants to lead us into repentance, and in order to do that we must admit to God that we have been wrong. It is often helpful to confess sins to a discreet confessor who loves God. (See pages 103–105 for the marks of a good confessor.)

3. Repentance. Repentance is not only feeling sorry for our sin; it is taking steps to avoid sinning in the future. Repentance includes making restitution where possible, apologizing, retracting statements when we have slandered, repaying what we have stolen, repairing what we have broken. Repentance means figuring out where we went wrong and how to avoid it the next time. If you had sex with your girlfriend or boyfriend, maybe next time you should not stay up until midnight cuddling alone. If you were gluttonous, maybe you need to keep sweets out of your house. If you were harsh with your spouse or children, maybe you need to get more sleep. Repentance especially means drawing on God's grace and strength, because our sins are forgiven through what Jesus did for us on the cross, and our lives are changed to the degree we allow Him to change us.

Spiritual health is more than just confessing our sins and altering bad behavior. It is also developing a new set of healthy behaviors.

Spending time with God is the basis of the Christian experience. Whatever else we do, we will never be successful as Christians if we do not spend intense time with God. We can do God's will and emulate His character only as much as we know Him. How do we get to know God?

Youthful fans of famous basketball players are careful to watch every game of their idol. They pore over the "stats" of their player (the statistics, if you don't have teenagers) and of every player on the team. They know what strategy he employs and how he overcomes his rivals on the field or court. The Christian should study his or her Bible just as assiduously, for this is the record of how God has acted in the past. It contains His game plan for the present and for the future. And it contains precious promises we can cling to.

If you are a serious basketball fan, you would jump at the chance to see your favorite team. Utter delight would include receiving your players' autographs, and ecstasy might include a few minutes talking with them. Christians have the great privilege and comfort of being able to talk to God at any time, to dwell in His presence. We can share our sorrow and our joys. We can request His guidance on any matter. We are even so privileged through the presence of the Holy Spirit in our lives as to get an occasional glimpse of heaven as God reveals Himself to us and acts through us. As we grow in God, we can learn how to open ourselves more fully to God and to be a better vessel of His love.

So far we have spoken only of our individual relationship with God. We do not have a relationship with God in a vacuum, however, because we were made to dwell in community; we have a corporate relationship with all believers. We need each other as a church community, and the church community needs us. Although we may find that we feel more "holy" when by ourselves, community life can be the fire that purifies us and keeps us humble.

When I was small I got a rock tumbler for my birthday. I was excited to select different stones and place them in the tumbler over several days with varying grades of sand. The abrasion of the sand and the constant friction of the other stones rubbed away the rough spots on the stones and eventually polished them to a finish almost like glass. So community life is with us. If we avoid our troubles (the sand) or the pressures of other personalities (the other stones), we may be more comfortable but we will be incomplete. Comfort is no indicator of Christian growth (Matthew 16:24), nor is it necessarily an indicator of emotional well-being.

Mark likes to write surrounded by radio talk shows or with the television on. He can tolerate the distraction of multiple phone calls or interruptions of all sorts. I, on the other hand, must have as close to absolute silence as I can get in an imperfect and noisy world. Part of our growth as individuals is accepting our differences. To me it is incredible that anyone can think coherently under the circumstances Mark writes, much less produce an intelligent article. To Mark it is unbelievable that I would want that much silence, much less require it.

The second (and more difficult) part of our growth is sacrificing our own desires and working in such a way as to accommodate each other (Ephesians 4:1–4). I often get up earlier than Mark, for instance, in order to have my silence. When he sees I am in the middle of a good writing session, he keeps his radio low and the TV off. I try to schedule my quiet sessions, on the other hand, when he is not around, knowing that silence (or, to me, relative quiet) is difficult for Mark to sustain. It is easier to be critical of each other's styles than to be sympathetic and supportive. But working toward a higher level, self-sacrifice, demonstrates a desire to grow in Christ and in our relationship with one another.

Let me be clear that not all compromise and self-sacrifice are of God. We can never condone what God has condemned. To pat someone on the back, for instance, and say it is O.K. to have sex outside of marriage is not loving. Love so cares about the other person that only God's will for that person is good enough. Tolerance will condone because it is based on seeking the other person's approval. (When we feel we must have other people's approval, incidentally, we are demonstrating some emotional damage and dysfunction that we should pay attention to and seek healing for.) Tolerance does not lie down and die for another person. Love does. We can never have corporate health as a Christian community if we try to substitute anemic tolerance for love just because it is more comfortable.

Few of the issues in the Christian community, on the other hand, are issues of right and wrong. Most of them (like the "best" writing environment) are matters of preference, the kinds of things we can compromise on. Recognizing the difference is an important step in Christian maturity.

In our search for wellness and health, we must sometimes accept discomfort. Spiritual and emotional health, like physical health, involve exercise and self-denial. But being healthy does not consist only of painful choices. Rather, it consists of reeducating ourselves to choose what is best for us. It is for this reason that our entire pursuit of health must be conducted under God's direction, for He alone knows what is best for us. In order to be well, we must walk in His ways.

Discussion Questions

1. Discuss several ways in which taking preventative measures physically, emotionally and spiritually is good stewardship.

2. Share your successes and failures in dieting.
3. What are some of the dietary and nutritional programs being recommended that are dubious, if not dangerous? What makes a program sound?
4. In recent years there have been numerous books, articles and television programs about the traits of a dysfunctional person, family or church. In what ways are these views compatible with biblical teaching? In what ways have they become the latest pop psychology or fad?
5. What are some of the roadblocks you have encountered in trying to spend regular quality time with the Lord? How did you work around those roadblocks?
6. In what ways are we actually unloving to people when we tolerate their sin?

Epilogue

God loves us, in deed as well as in word. He who did not spare His only Son, but gave Him up for our redemption, continues to make available His blessings to us at our points of need—and that includes healing of body, soul and spirit. He does not give these blessings reluctantly or grudgingly. His desire to bless is greater than our desire to be blessed! As we are healed, we enter more fully into our heritage as His sons and daughters, we grow closer to Him in love, gratitude and obedience, and we are motivated and equipped to serve the world in His name (see John 21:15–17). What a privilege!

The extraordinary thing is that God has chosen to carry on His work of healing through ordinary folk like ourselves. Empowered by His grace, led by His Spirit, instructed by His Word and submitted to His elders, we can be used to accomplish His purposes. The result? God's name is glorified, His people are blessed, His Church is edified and His Kingdom is extended.

My prayer for all who read this book is that you will be made whole and that you will minister this wholeness to others.

Being Overcome by the Power of the Holy Spirit

A phenomenon sometimes encountered in a service of healing is that of people falling over backwards when someone prays for them. Popularly referred to as "being slain in the Spirit," it is not the same as fainting. The person has not lost consciousness. Rather, he or she is coming into a state of great peace and, often, close fellowship with God. A person may rest in this state for a few minutes or for more than an hour.

As with any other spiritual experience, it is authentic and helpful when it is a work of God, but harmful and destructive when people are manipulated, worked up emotionally or deliberately pushed over. The presence or absence of this phenomenon neither validates nor discredits either the person ministering or the person being ministered to—unless there is a deliberate attempt to force it to happen or to block it from happening. In the former case, people can become disillusioned about the movement of the Holy Spirit in general. In the latter case, a blessing from God might be thrown away and one of the vehicles for healing set aside. In short, we are neither to force it nor prevent it.

Possible scriptural references to this phenomenon are Acts 9:4, where we are told Saul was knocked to the ground by a powerful intervention of God, and John 18:6, where we read that the Roman soldiers fell to the ground. This group was not falling at the feet of Jesus to worship Him, nor were these strong, tough men shrinking back in fear. Rather, at this moment of betrayal, when the stage was set for the Son of God to go to the cross to make atonement for human sin, the presence and power of God must have been so strong that the soldiers could not stand.

There are many references to this experience throughout the history of the Church. I have chosen just three to illustrate how this experience is neither new nor the property only of Pentecostal groups. Notice that the references come from different centuries, different countries, different denominations and different places on what might be called the ecclesiastical ladder.

First, St. Teresa of Avila, a sixteenth-century Spanish Roman Catholic nun. She wrote this about the phenomenon:

> The soul becomes conscious that it is fainting almost completely away, in a kind of swoon, with an exceeding great and sweet delight. It gradually ceases to breathe and all its bodily strength begins to fail it. . . . He can apprehend nothing with the senses, which only hinder his soul's joy and thus harm rather than help him. It is futile for him to attempt to speak: his mind cannot form a single word, nor, if it could, would he have the strength to pronounce it. For in this condition all outward strength vanishes, while the strength of the soul increases so that it may have the fruition of its bliss. The outward joy experienced is great and most clearly recognized.

Second, George Whitefield, eighteenth-century English Anglican (Episcopalian) priest. The following account was given of what happened at a large outdoor service at which Whitefield was the speaker:

> Some were struck pale as death, others were wringing their hands, others lying on the ground, others were sinking into the arms of their friends.

Third, Charles G. Finney, nineteenth-century American Presbyterian layman (and lawyer by trade). The following account was given by Finney of a service he was leading in Utica, New York. The circumstances of those being overcome by the Holy Spirit were not, he commented,

cases of . . . objectionable excitement. . . . . Manifestly there is no such effervescence of the sensibility as produces tears, or any of the usual manifestations of an excited imagination, or deeply moved feelings. There is not that gush of feeling which distracts the thoughts; but the mind sees truth, unveiled and in such relations as really to take away all bodily strength, while the mind looks in upon the unveiled glories of the Godhead. The veil seems to be removed from the mind, and the truth is seen much as we suppose it to be when the spirit is disembodied. No wonder this should overpower the body.

What is God's purpose in causing people to be overcome by the power of the Holy Spirit? Those who have experienced it testify that it is an occasion of blessing. Many speak of spiritual and emotional refreshment. Some receive healing—especially, but not exclusively, of a spiritual or emotional kind. Some sense God speaking to them. Some receive visions. Some liken the inner cleansing that occurs to a "spiritual sauna." A reasonable hypothesis is that this experience provides a moment of rest when one's customary defenses and controls are lowered and one becomes more receptive to the Lord's activity. God can use the experience, too, to gain a person's attention, to let him know the reality of divine power.

There are many different ways in which falling under the power of the Spirit happens. Some people fall straight back, smoothly and easily. Others seem to resist what is happening, stop, step back a bit to catch themselves and then drop suddenly. Others drop straight down into a heap. Occasionally someone falls forward into the one praying for him. People can experience this phenomenon even at a distance from the person praying for them. It can happen to a person individually or as part of a group. Often one is "slain" in response to the laying on of hands, or by being touched with holy water, anointing oil or similar sacramentals.

In the service I led for several years in Malden, Massachusetts, we gave the title "catcher" to those whose primary task was to stand behind persons being prayed for in case they should come under the power of the Holy Spirit. The catcher's job was to lower them to the floor so they would not be hurt. Some do not see the need for a catcher, believing that God will not allow a person to be hurt by falling over when He pours the Spirit down upon him or her. While this is often true, it is not *always* true. The fact is, I have seen people hurt and have heard of this happening from others. Just as Jesus would not tempt His Father by jumping from the pinnacle of the Temple (although I believe that had Jesus slipped and fallen, the angels would have caught Him), we should refuse to tempt God by not providing a catcher.

Robert Shelton, who served as our trainer and supervisor of catchers, has offered this helpful advice on what to do if you are ever called upon to be a catcher:

> There is an art to catching and it is easily learned. Never attempt to hold a person up, because the person "slain" becomes dead weight and awkward to hold. Catch the person under the armpits and step backward so that you may lay the person out flat without dropping or hurting him. Try never to drop a person on his buttocks since this could lead to a nasty injury to the coccyx bone at the base of the spine.
>
> While lowering the person, be careful of your own back. Remember to use your arm and leg muscles and not your back muscles when you are lowering someone.
>
> Be aware of the clothing that people are wearing, for several reasons. One, silky clothing makes it hard to hold people. They could slip from your grasp. Two, be aware of the state of the person's clothing so that there is no embarrassment when he or she is at rest on the floor. Three, be careful not to damage the clothing; tearing is possible.
>
> Remember one more thing: The catcher is also one of the prayers for the relief or healing of the person. You have as much input to the person as the rest of the team. You might pray in silence or aloud just like the rest of the team.
>
> Good catching, and be careful!

Once people have been overcome by the Spirit and safely settled on the floor, we have found it unwise to attempt to rush them back to their feet. For one thing, this might be difficult, as they are in a physically unstable state. More importantly, to get them up too soon would interrupt whatever it is that God is trying to do. Until such point as they try to get onto their feet, the whole team, or one team member detached for this purpose, should continue to pray alongside them. This prayer, however, should be very quiet. I have experienced occasions when I could not hear what God was trying to say to me because the team members were praying too loudly over me. When the people on the floor attempt to get to their feet, help them, remembering to bend your knees so as not to hurt your back. Notice whether they are sufficiently recovered to get back to their seats without further help, and, if not, offer them that help.

A Diagnostic Checklist

The following checklist has been prepared to help you find possible causes of an illness and in keeping good physical-emotional-spiritual health for yourself and those to whom you minister. The fact that this list is lengthy should serve as a warning to avoid simplistic judgments as to why a person is sick. To assist yourself and others in coming to and maintaining health, an honest, Holy Spirit-assisted use of this list on a regular basis is strongly suggested.

A. Physical Condition
  1. Do you maintain a balanced diet of basic food groups?
  2. Do you take in too many or too few calories on a regular basis?
  3. Have you been checked for nutritional deficiency in a particular mineral? For allergies?
  4. What is the amount and quality of your sleep?
  5. What is the amount and regularity of your exercise?
  6. Do you smoke? Do you drink more than eight ounces of wine, two beers or two mixed drinks each day? Do you use any other "social drug"?
  7. Has there been a recent occurrence of physical trauma—that is, a fall, strain, bump, accident?
  8. Do you regularly have physical, dental and eye examinations?

9. Are there hereditary illnesses, conditions?
10. Have you been chaste/monogamous? If you are married, has your spouse?
11. Are you on any medications? Do you take them as prescribed?

B. Spiritual Practice
1. Do you read the Bible each day? Do you submit to what God tells you to believe?
2. Do you try, with God's help, to live an obedient life, surrendering control of your will to God and seeking to bring your actions into conformity with God's will?
3. Do you pray regularly? Does your prayer life include several modes of prayer such as adoration, meditation, confession, intercession, petition? Do you take time to be still in God's presence?
4. Do you worship regularly with other Christians?
5. Do you have regular fellowship with other Christians?
6. Do you receive regular individual spiritual direction or guidance?
7. Do you confess your sins to God regularly, either directly or to another person? Are you too hard on yourself? Too easy? Do you find it difficult to accept God's forgiveness? Do you want to be forgiven but are unwilling to change? Do you let God examine your whole life or do you hold some things back? Do you forgive others?
8. Do you regularly receive holy Communion?
9. Do you have a good balance of emphasis in your spiritual practice among doctrine (study of Scripture and Christian books), discipline (obedience to God's commands), devotion (adoration, praise, worship, meditation, silence before God)?
10. Are you trying to grow spiritually in your own strength or are you asking God to grow you through grace?
11. Is your spirituality authentically yours (God makes

people with different spiritualities, temperaments)
or are you trying to be like someone else?

12. Most importantly, are you trusting Christ as your
hope for heaven, or are you "trusting in your own
righteousness"?

C. Psychological/Emotional Health
  1. Past
     a. Are there people, places or periods of your life
        that you have blotted out or that you avoid or
        deny?
     b. Does the recollection of certain people, places,
        events produce great feelings of shame, guilt,
        fear, hurt, anger or rejection?
  2. Present
     a. Are there recurrent problems with social inter-
        actions, close relationships?
     b. Are you afraid to be alone? Do you always want
        to be alone? Can you be by yourself and enjoy it
        (solitude vs. loneliness)? Do you enjoy only
        being by yourself and not being with others?
     c. Are you constantly dependent on others to vali-
        date or approve you? Do you accept yourself?
     d. Are you afraid to share intimate inner knowl-
        edge with anyone? Do you share too readily,
        indiscriminately?
     e. Are there things you should be able to do that
        you cannot do, for reasons that are difficult to
        articulate?
     f. Can you be assertive (standing up for your
        rights while respecting those of others) or are
        you generally passive or aggressive?
     g. Do you have violent mood swings?
     h. Are you happy with who you are while
        acknowledging and acting on the need for
        improvement?
     i. Do you compare yourself favorably or unfavor-
        ably to others?
     j. Do you always go along with the group? Always
        insist on your own way? (That is to say, are you

a compulsive "people-pleaser" or one who is
rigid and inflexible?)

k. Do you generally make yourself the focus of
attention/subject of conversation (whether
positively or negatively)? Or do you avoid being
the topic of discussion at all costs?

l. How do you deal with criticism? Do you automatically disagree/defend yourself or agree/put
yourself down?

m. Do you generally resolve arguments by giving
in? By trying to win at all costs?

3. Future

a. Are you anxious and fearful about the future?

b. Do you have goals for the future that are realistic for your age, gifts, background? Are you
making steady progress toward those goals? Are
you able to reassess and redefine goals when
appropriate? Do you live from crisis to crisis?

c. Does your existence consist of "hours of boredom, moments of panic"?

D. Occult Involvement

1. Is or was there involvement by your parents or
grandparents in witchcraft or the occult?

2. Have you ever been involved in occult or New Age
practices? (See Appendix 5 for a list of these.) If so,
have you renounced them?

3. Is it particularly difficult for you to pray, praise God
in worship, receive ministry, honor the name of
Jesus?

4. Do you feel more than a normal compulsion to do
wrong things? To take the Lord's name in vain?

5. Do you feel as though you have one or more extra
personalities within you?

6. Do you hear voices or have dreams that are generally terrifying or hostile?

Healings Recorded in Scripture

Healings in the Old Testament

1. Abimelech healed; Abimelech's wife and female slaves healed of barrenness.	Genesis 20:1–18
2. Abraham's wife Sarah healed of barrenness.	Genesis 21:1–7
3. Moses healed of leprosy at the burning bush.	Exodus 4:1–7
4. Moses' sister, Miriam, healed of leprosy.	Numbers 12:1–15
5. Moses successfully stops a plague.	Numbers 16:41–50
6. Snakebites healed in the wilderness.	Numbers 21:4–9
7. Manoah's wife healed of barrenness.	Judges 13:2–24
8. King Jeroboam's paralyzed hand healed by "a man of God."	1 Kings 13:1–6
9. Elijah restores to life a widow's son.	1 Kings 17:17–24
10. Elisha restores to life the son of a Shunammite woman.	2 Kings 4:8–37
11. Elisha heals Naaman of leprosy.	2 Kings 5:1–14
12. Isaiah heals King Hezekiah of a boil and prolongs his life.	2 Kings 20:1–11; Isaiah 38:1–8
13. Job healed of leprosy and of various losses.	Job 2:7–8; 42:10–16

Healings by Jesus in the New Testament

1. Multitudes healed and delivered at Galilee.	Matthew 4:23; Mark 1:39; Luke 6:17–19
2. Leper healed.	Matthew 8:1–4; Mark 1:40–42; Luke 5:12–15
3. Centurion's servant healed of paralysis.	Matthew 8:5–13; Luke 7:2–10
4. Peter's mother-in-law healed of a fever.	Matthew 8:14–15; Mark 1:30–31; Luke 4:38–39
5. Multitudes healed and delivered from demons.	Matthew 8:16–17; Mark 1:32–34; Luke 4:40–41
6. Gadarene demoniacs delivered.	Matthew 8:28–34; Mark 5:1–15; Luke 8:26–33
7. Paralytic man healed and forgiven.	Matthew 9:2–8; Mark 2:3–12; Luke 5:17–26
8. Jairus' daughter restored to life.	Matthew 9:18–19, 23–25; Mark 5:22–24, 35–43; Luke 8:41–42, 49–56
9. Woman healed of hemorrhage.	Matthew 9:20–22; Mark 5:25–34; Luke 8:43–48
10. Two blind men healed.	Matthew 9:27–30
11. Mute, demon-possessed man healed and delivered.	Matthew 9:32–33

12. Multitudes healed.	Matthew 9:35
13. Healings cited to convince John the Baptist that Jesus was the Messiah.	Luke 7:19–22
14. Man with a withered hand healed on the Sabbath.	Matthew 12:10–13; Mark 3:1–5; Luke 6:6–10
15. Multitudes healed near Capernaum.	Matthew 12:15; Mark 3:9–11
16. Blind, mute, demon-possessed man healed and delivered.	Matthew 12:22; Luke 11:14
17. Multitudes healed in the desert right before Jesus fed the 5,000.	Matthew 14:13–14; Luke 9:11; John 6:2
18. Multitudes healed at Gennesaret as they touched the fringe of Jesus' garment.	Matthew 14:34–36; Mark 6:55–56
19. Daughter of Syrophoenician woman delivered.	Matthew 15:22–28; Mark 7:24–30
20. Multitudes healed on a mountain near the Sea of Galilee.	Matthew 15:29–31
21. Epileptic boy healed, delivered.	Matthew 17:14–18; Mark 9:14–27; Luke 9:38–43
22. Multitudes healed in Judea beyond the Jordan River.	Matthew 19:1–2
23. Two blind men healed near Jericho.	Matthew 20:29–34
24. Blind and lame people healed in the Temple.	Matthew 21:12–14
25. Man with an unclean spirit delivered.	Mark 1:22–26; Luke 4:33–36
26. A few in Nazareth healed.	Mark 6:5

27. Deaf and mute man healed.	Mark 7:31–35
28. Blind man at Bethsaida healed.	Mark 8:22–26
29. Blind Bartimaeus healed.	Mark 10:46–52; Luke 18:35–43
30. Multitudes gather to be healed after Jesus healed the leper.	Luke 5:15
31. Young man at Nain restored to life.	Luke 7:11–16
32. Bent-over woman with a spirit of infirmity healed.	Luke 13:11–16
33. Man with dropsy healed.	Luke 14:1–4
34. Ten lepers healed.	Luke 17:11–19
35. Severed ear of Malchus healed at Gethsemane.	Luke 22:50–51
36. Nobleman's son healed.	John 4:46–53
37. Infirm man at Bethesda healed.	John 5:2–15
38. Man blind from birth healed.	John 9:1–11
39. Lazarus restored to life.	John 11:1–44
40. Jesus raised from death by God the Father.	Matthew 28:1–10; Mark 16:1–14; Luke 24:1–43; John 20:1–29

Healings through the Disciples of Jesus

1. Internship of the Twelve.	Matthew 10:1–8; Mark 3:13–19; 6:7–13; Luke 9:1
2. Internship of the seventy.	Luke 10:1–9
3. The apostles perform signs and wonders on the Day of Pentecost.	Acts 2:43
4. Peter and John minister healing to a man lame from birth.	Acts 3:1–16
5. The apostles perform signs and wonders in Solomon's Portico.	Acts 5:12–16

6. Philip casts out demons and ministers healing to paralyzed and lame people in Samaria.	Acts 8:5–7
7. Ananias ministers healing to Saul (Paul) for his blindness.	Acts 9:10–19
8. Peter ministers healing to the paralyzed Aeneas at Lydda.	Acts 9:32–34
9. Peter is used to restore Tabitha (Dorcas) to life at Joppa.	Acts 9:36–41
10. Paul and Barnabas minister by signs and wonders.	Acts 14:3
11. Paul ministers healing to a crippled man at Lystra.	Acts 14:8–10
12. Paul casts out evil spirit from a young woman at Thyatira.	Acts 16:16–18
13. Healings and deliverances ministered by Paul at Ephesus.	Acts 19:11–12
14. Eutychus restored to life through Paul's prayers.	Acts 20:7–12
15. Paul is healed from venomous viper bite at Malta.	Acts 28:1–6
16. Paul ministers healing at Malta to the father of Publius, who suffers from a fever and dysentery.	Acts 28:7–8
17. Other people on Malta are healed through the ministry of Paul.	Acts 28:9

Study Questions about Scripture Passages on Healing

The Facts of the Incident

1. Describe the person in need (including age, sex, social status).
2. What was the apparent need?
    a. How was this expressed by the person involved?
    b. How was it expressed by others?
3. What was being sought? By whom?
4. Did Jesus say what the cause of the person's problem was? If yes, what was the cause?
5. Who took the initiative in effecting a healing?
    a. The person in need? If so, how?
    b. Others? If so, how?
    c. Jesus? If so, how?
6. Processes involved leading to healing:
    a. What did Jesus say?
    b. What did Jesus do?
    c. What did Jesus tell the person in need to do?
    d. What did Jesus tell the others to do?
7. Reactions to the healing:
    a. How did the person in need react?

b. How did the others react?
c. Did Jesus say anything about the healing after it was accomplished, and, if so, what?

Your Personal Evaluation

1. After reading the record, what do you think was the matter with the person in need?
2. Attitude toward ministry:
    a. What was the attitude of Jesus concerning a ministry of healing to the person in need?
    b. What was the attitude of others concerning the possibility of healing?
    c. What was the attitude of the person in need?
3. The place of faith and love in effecting a restoration to health:
    a. What attitude does Jesus tell the person in need he will have to assume if he expects to be healed?
    b. Did the person in need give any verbal expression of faith?
    c. Did any others give any verbal expression of faith?
    d. Identify all nonverbal evidences of faith in the narrative.
    e. How did Jesus manifest His faith or express His love?
4. What were the evidences of healing?
5. Why do you think Jesus performed this healing?

These study questions are from the
Order of St. Luke and used with
gratitude.

Appendix 5

Statements and Prayers

A Statement of Dedication or Rededication to Christ as Lord and Savior

Heavenly Father, I admit to You that I am a sinner. I have sinned in thought, word and deed, and by what I have failed to do. I acknowledge that I cannot earn my salvation but need Jesus to be my Savior. I know that He died on the cross to pay the penalty for my sins. I now ask Jesus to be my Savior and to take away the penalty of my sins, so that I can have fellowship with You, both now and in heaven. Thank You, Jesus, for being my Savior. By Your grace I wish to live in conformity to Your will and make You the Lord of my life. Amen.

A Prayer of Confession of Sin

Heavenly Father, I acknowledge that I have sinned in thought, word, deed, and by failure to do that which You have called me to do. In particular I acknowledge my sins of _____, I acknowledge my ongoing orientation of _____ and I admit my fascination with _____. Lord God, I know these things are wrong and I ask Your forgiveness. I thank You that Jesus paid the penalty for my sins at Calvary and His blood can

319

wash me from my sins. I claim His atoning work for me right now. And I ask the Holy Spirit to give me grace to turn from these sins, orientations and fascinations, that I may live from now on in holiness of life. Through Jesus Christ, my Lord and Savior. Amen.

(In the blanks you may add specific sins and orientations that are not in keeping with the will of God, and fascination with actions, attitudes or orientations that are not of God.)

A Statement of Renunciation of Occult Practice

Lord Jesus Christ, I acknowledge that there are spiritual powers in the universe that are in rebellion against You. Through my ignorance and willfulness I have given these a place in my life. I have called out to various "spiritual powers." I have participated in spiritual practices You have forbidden, such as _____. I turn my back on them and renounce any place they have in my life. I command, in the name of the Lord Jesus Christ and in the power of the cross, that any spiritual entities not submitted to God leave me. I ask the Holy Spirit to come and fill any place in my spirit made empty by their departure. And I ask, Lord Jesus Christ, that You give me grace to live only for You and to be kept steadfast in my walk with You. Through Jesus Christ, my Lord and Master. Amen.

(In the blank mention any involvement in the worship of, devotion to, calling out to or following of any spiritual entity other than the God of Scripture; or any involvement in such occult practices as tarot cards, ouija boards, meditation that is not the historic Christian kind of meditation, séances, contacting the dead, palmreading, water-witching, mindreading, channeling, magic [other than sleight of hand or card tricks], use of crystals for healing or magic purposes, casting spells, using a crystal ball, manufacturing or using magic potions, astrology, etc.)

A Statement of Renunciation of Satan and of Commitment to Jesus Christ as Lord and Savior

Question: Do you renounce Satan and all the spiritual forces of wickedness that rebel against God?

Answer: I renounce them.

Question: Do you renounce the evil powers of this world that
              corrupt and destroy the creatures of God?

Answer: I renounce them.

Question: Do you renounce all sinful desires that draw you
              from the love of God?

Answer: I renounce them.

Question: Do you turn to Jesus Christ and accept Him as your
              Savior?

Answer: I do.

Question: Do you put your whole trust in His grace and love?

Answer: I do.

Question: Do you promise to follow and obey Him as your
              Lord?

Answer: I do.

Service of Holy Baptism
Book of Common Prayer
pages 302–303

Several Forms of Exorcism

Exorcism of persons

You evil spirit, I command you in the name of the Lord Jesus
Christ and by His cross and precious blood to depart from this person. I command you to go directly to Jesus for your future fate,
and I forbid you to harm anyone along the way. Lord Jesus Christ,
please fill with the Holy Spirit the places in [name] now made empty
by the departing of these evil spirits. Amen.

* * * * * * *

I exorcise you, every unclean spirit, in the Name of God the
Father Almighty, in the Name of Jesus Christ His Son and our Lord
and our Judge, and by the Power of the Holy Spirit, to be gone
from this image of God [name] whom our Lord in His goodness
has called to His Holy Temple, that he [she] himself [herself] may
become a temple of the Living God, and the Holy Spirit may dwell

in him [her]. Through the same Christ our Lord Who will come to judge the living and the dead and the world by fire. Amen.

from the *Rituale Romanum*

Exorcism of places

Deliver, O Lord, this place [or house, dwelling, church] from all presence of the evil one, all evil spirits, all noises, feelings, senses, phantasms and presences. Make them depart from here and go to the place you have assigned them, never to return. Bring peace to this place, O Lord, and fill it with Your presence. Through Jesus Christ, our Lord. Amen.

* * * * * * *

Pour Your blessing on this place [or house, dwelling, church] and make it a place set apart for You. Drive far from it, O Lord, the presence of any spirit not submitted to You. In Your mercy, place Your warrior angels as a hedge to guard and defend all in this place [or house, dwelling, church] and keep us safe from the evil one and all his minions. Indwell it, Holy Spirit, that all who enter [or enter and dwell, or enter and worship] here may be drawn closer in knowledge, faith and love to You, the Father and our Lord Jesus Christ. May the Lord bless and sanctify this tabernacle of His servants and grant them the riches of the Kingdom of heaven. In Jesus' name. Amen.

Commendation of the Soul of a Dead Person

Of the soul of someone known to have died in the faith of Christ

Into thy hands, O merciful Savior, we commend thy servant [name]. Acknowledge, we humbly beseech thee, a sheep of thine own flock, a sinner of thine own redeeming. Receive *him* into the arms of thy mercy, into the blessed rest of everlasting peace, and into the glorious company of the saints in light. *Amen.*

The Book of Common Prayer, p. 483

Of the soul whose faith is known to God alone

We commend, O merciful Lord, the soul of [name], departed. We commend him [her] to Your merciful and wise judgment, knowing that Your judgment is true. Through Jesus Christ our Lord. Amen.

Clinical Evidence
for Healing

Positive Therapeutic Effects of Intercessory Prayer in a Coronary Care Unit Population

Randolph C. Byrd, M.D., San Francisco, California

Abstract: The therapeutic effects of intercessory prayer (IP) to the Judeo-Christian God, one of the oldest forms of therapy, has had little attention in the medical literature. To evaluate the effects of IP in a coronary care unit (CCU) population, a prospective randomized double-blind protocol was followed. Over ten months, 393 patients admitted to the CCU were randomized, after signing informed consent, to an intercessory prayer group (192 patients) or to a control group (201 patients). While hospitalized, the first group received IP by participating Christians praying outside the hospital; the control group did not. At entry, chi-square and stepwise logistic analysis revealed no statistical difference between the groups. After entry, all patients had follow-up for the remainder of the admission. The IP group subsequently had a significantly lower severity score based on the hospital course after entry ($P < .01$). Multivariant analysis separated the groups on the basis of the outcome variables ($P < .0001$). The control patients required ventilatory assistance, antibiotics, and diuretics more frequently than patients in the IP group. These data suggest that intercessory prayer to the Judeo-Christian God has a beneficial therapeutic effect in patients admitted to a CCU.

For the complete article, please see pp. 826–829 of the July 1988 issue of the *Southern Medical Journal.*

ॐ

The question is often raised why, despite the large percentage of the population claiming faith in God, there is a limited number of clinical studies relating the impact of religion on objective health measures. One reason may be funding. Pharmaceutical companies fund research experiments because positive outcomes are necessary for approval of their products. Few religious organizations have the resources to devote to such studies. Another reason may be residual effects of the so-called Enlightenment period. "Scientists of that era flushed with enthusiasm for their new discoveries, wished and needed to unshackle themselves from the church. . . . The burgeoning successes of the scientific method created new tensions in the relationship between religion and medicine, leading eventually to a split in which religion was forced to restrict itself to the role of caretaker of the soul, while the role of medicine became that of caretaker of the body, and later, the mind. Faith, by its very nature, was deemed to be unobjective and not verifiable, and hence, unscientific and not worthy of data-based research."

From the introduction to
"The Faith Factor: An Annotated Bibliography of
Clinical Research on Spiritual Subjects,"
by Dale A. Matthews, M.D.,
David B. Larson, M.D., M.S.P.H.,
and Constance P. Barry, M.P.H.

This two-volume study is the best collection of summaries of articles from various research journals on the relationship between religion (or faith) and physical and emotional health. For further information, consult the publishers: National Institute for Healthcare Research, One Colonial Pl., 2111 Wilson Blvd., Suite 1130, Arlington, VA 22201.

ॐ

What follows are citations of a few of the articles from the research literature.

1. A study on "The Impact of Religion on Men's Blood Pressure" noted that the self-perceived importance of religion was directly associated with lower blood pressure. *Journal of Religion and Health* 1989; 28:265–278.

2. The study "Religious Belief, Depression and Ambulation Status in Elderly Women with Broken Hips" found that belief in God and frequency of church attendance was significantly related to post-operative ambulation status and inversely correlated with level of depression in the study group. *American Journal of Psychiatry* 1990; 147:758–760.

3. A study of nearly 100,000 people noted that frequency of church attendance is associated with significant reductions in morbidity and mortality from a variety of disease conditions. *Journal of Chronic Diseases* 1972; 25:665–672.

4. "The Effect of Prayer on Well-Being" in *Journal of Psychology and Theology* 1991; 19(1):71–83 notes a strong and positive correlation of religious practice with multiple measures of well-being.

5. Religious commitment is positively associated with psychological adjustment and life satisfaction according to the study "The Relationship Between Religion and Mental Health/Distress," published in *Review of Religious Research* 1989; 31(1):16–22.

6. The article "Does Religion Influence Adult Health?" noted that the greater the practice of one's religion, the better one's health. *Journal for the Scientific Study of Religion* 1991; 30(2):193–202.

7. Religious commitment and prayer for healing were demonstrated to produce long-term success for those quitting smoking in the study "Factors Determining the Success of Nicotine Withdrawal: 12-Year Follow-up of 532 Smokers After Suggestion Therapy (by a Faith Healer)," published in *The International Journal of the Addictions* 1987; 22(12): 1189–1200.

8. The article "Frequency of Church Attendance and Blood Pressure Elevation" demonstrated that frequency of church

attendance is inversely related to blood pressure regardless of age, sex, socioeconomic status and body mass. *Journal of Behavioral Medicine* 1978; 1:37–43.

9. High religious involvement is associated positively with lower rates of alcohol and drug abuse among those with mood disorders in the study "Alcohol and Drug Abuse in Patients with Affective Syndromes." *Comprehensive Psychiatry* 1985; 26(3):283–295.

10. Religious orthodoxy is often attacked for the harm it is believed to cause individuals. The study "Relationship Between Religious Orthodoxy and Three Mental Health Factors" demonstrated, however, that religious orthodoxy was negatively correlated with hostility and had no negative associations with a person's anxiety or self-esteem. *Psychological Reports* 1976; 38:756–758.

11. Orthodox religious belief and practice is correlated positively with greater life satisfaction in older people in the study "Religion, Age, Life Satisfaction, and Perceived Sources of Religiousness: A Study of Older Persons." *Journal of Gerontology* 1985; 40(5):615–20.

12. Sometimes those hostile to religion assert that religious commitment is a, if not the, cause of psychopathology. The study "Psychopathology and Religious Commitment" demonstrated, however, that mental illness and the strength of religious commitment are inversely related. *Review of Religious Research* 1971; 12(3):165–175.

13. A lengthy article in *Prevention in Human Services* (1991; 9:41–64) reviews various research articles on the relationship between religious practice and physical health. The authors, J. S. Levin and H. Y. Vanderpool, demonstrate how, in various ways, faith has a generally beneficial role.

14. Another article that reviews various studies is "Religious Domains and General Well-Being," published in *Social Indicators Research* 1989; 22:1–22. Authors M. M. Poloma and B. F. Pendleton note how religious commitment and general well-being are positively associated.

The Service
of Holy Communion
as a Service of Healing

Many of us have been to a healing service. But do you realize that every service of holy Communion is a healing service? In this section we will look at the various parts of the Communion service and how they relate to the ministry of Christian healing. It is my hope that every time you are at a service of holy Communion, you can find in it a means to your healing—physical, emotional and spiritual.

Opening Acts of Praise

Nearly every Communion service, unless it is a quiet early Sunday morning or a daytime midweek service, begins with a hymn. In many churches, especially those touched by the renewal movement, there are several songs of praise. Such acts of praise serve to get us in touch with God, who dwells in the praises of His people (Psalm 22:3, KJV). Besides opening us to God, praise serves to strengthen our faith. Our orientation is upward, toward Him from whom all blessings flow, and away from ourselves, giving God the freedom to work in us and helping us to get out of the way. Our thoughts can focus on the words of the music, which often build

328

our faith by describing who God is, how much He loves us and what He does. Often, long before specific prayers for our needs, God intervenes when, as the song says, we "forget about ourselves and concentrate on Him."

The Ministry of the Word

In most Communion services, the time of praise is followed by a time of reading from the Scriptures and a sermon based on them. This relates to Christian healing in at least two ways.

1. As we hear about the promises of God. God makes many promises to us and the reading of Scripture reminds us of them. Some lessons tell us specifically about God's promises of healing; other readings remind us of other promises. Even though the promises may not specifically relate to healing, we are reminded— by statements of promise and by stories of how those promises were received over the centuries by His people in need—that God offers us His very best. Confident that God wants to bless us, we can approach Him with our needs of the present.

2. As we hear about the commands of God. God calls us to discipleship, lived out as we bring before Him all aspects of our life. Much spiritual sickness comes because of our sin. When we sin, we place a barrier between ourselves and God, and our relationship with God suffers. Although not all physical or emotional sickness happens because of our sin, some does, as we have already seen.

When we hear what God expects of us as the Word of God is read and preached, we have an opportunity for repentance, for receiving divine forgiveness, for coming into restoration of fellowship with God and for healing.

The Recitation of the Creed

The Creed, either the Apostles' Creed or the Nicene Creed, is a summary statement of the basics of the Christian faith. We may not understand every part of it, but in reciting the Creed we are saying that we acknowledge the truths God has given us. Unless we consider ourselves above God and above the collective wisdom of the Church throughout the centuries, we will never pick and choose among the articles of the Creed, believing only what we wish. Our attitude must always be, "This is what You have revealed, Lord. I receive it by faith. Please help me understand what it means and apply it to my life."

The Creed relates to healing in this way: It points us to God and away from any of the other spiritual beings in the universe. Many of these spiritual beings are in open rebellion to God, and our relating to them, whether intentionally or by a lazy, fuzzy understanding of who God is, can be very harmful, even though initially it may even bring a measure of healing. In this day of increased Satanism, New Age occultism and so-called alternative Christian spiritualities, a proper understanding of who God is (and is not) is very important.

The Prayers of the People

During the time of congregational prayer, we have an opportunity to pray for the needs of the world, the Church, other people and ourselves. In many churches a list of names of sick parishioners is read. In some churches this list is reproduced in the Sunday bulletin for people to take home and use in daily devotions.

In some churches opportunity is given for people to speak prayer concerns aloud. At least half of the specific accounts in the Gospels of Jesus ministering healing describe Him as healing people in response to the intercession of others. What an opportunity to take to the throne of grace the needs of loved ones, and to do it with the prayer support of our fellow worshipers! When praying aloud for someone during a church service, therefore, make sure you speak loudly enough that you can be heard by others.

Confession and Absolution

One of the causes of our physical, emotional and spiritual sickness, as we saw earlier, is our own sin. The time of the confession in the Communion service is a time to acknowledge our sins before the Lord so that they can be forgiven and their consequences removed.

We should never rely *solely* on such general confession. The liturgical formula for confession is, by necessity, general and brief. Our time of doing real business with the Lord is beforehand. The liturgical formula of some churches, however, is a helpful reminder that we have already confessed and can approach God with our needs with our guilt taken away. Sometimes it serves as a reminder of what we yet need to do.

Absolution is a time when God's ministers pronounce forgiveness in His name to those who want to turn from their sins. It is a good reminder that "if we confess our sins, he is faithful and just, and will forgive our sins and cleanse us from all unrighteousness" (1 John 1:9). Satan is the "accuser of our brethren" (Revelation 12:10) and will try to get us to believe that our sins are such that God will never forgive us, much less bless or heal us. The absolution is a good reminder that what Jesus did on Calvary is sufficient atonement for sin. If we confess with purpose of amendment of life, God forgives, no matter what Satan may say or what thoughts he may try to put into our consciences.

Some clergy, in pronouncing absolution, make the sign of the cross over the people. This is a wonderful visual reminder that between our sins and the just judgment of God stands the atoning, forgiving cross of Christ. Many people—not just Roman Catholics, Eastern Orthodox or Episcopalians—make the sign of the cross over themselves as an acknowledgment of what Christ has done in forgiving our sins.

The Exchange of the Peace

In many orders of service, right after the absolution comes the exchange of the peace. (In the Roman Catholic liturgy this occurs immediately before the people come forward to receive Communion.) "Passing the peace"—in some churches simply a time of greeting one another—is a reminder that while Christianity is a *personal* relationship with God, it is not a *private* one. That is to say, while we are to have a one-on-one relationship with God, we are also to have, in Christ, relationships with other Christians. There is no such thing as solo Christianity.

During the exchange of the peace we may discover we are not comfortable greeting certain individuals. In fact, we may find ourselves trying to figure out how we can greet our friends while avoiding the embarrassing situation of having to exchange the peace with certain others. This could be God's way of telling us that there is some work of reconciliation yet to be done, either right then or soon after. We are not required to have every member of the church as our close friend or to agree with them on everything. We *are* called to be at peace with them, insofar as it lies within us (Romans 14:19; Hebrews 12:14). To be at enmity with another person often manifests itself in spiritual, emotional or even physical sickness.

The Offertory

For many of us the offertory is simply a time to put our offering envelope in the plate and sit back and listen to an anthem from the choir. It is, however, much more than that. The money we place in the plate is not our dues for belonging to the organization. It represents the offering of our whole selves—our treasure, yes, but also our time, our talents, our very being. We are not giving God money to buy favors from Him. We are surrendering ourselves to God, who gives His blessings as grace—free and unmerited favor. We are reminded of this in the words of the Doxology sung in many churches: "Praise God from whom all blessings flow." In other churches these words are said or sung: "All things come of Thee, O Lord, and of Thine own have we given Thee."

The Prayer of Consecration

There are at least two ways in which the prayer consecrating (or setting apart) the Communion elements relates to the ministry of healing.

1. It reminds us of what Christ did for us on Calvary. On Calvary Jesus offered His life in atonement for sin. Because of our sin we are estranged from God—a spiritual sickness of the first order. Our lostness makes us susceptible to various other bad fruits of human fallenness—emotional and physical sickness. On the cross Jesus paid the penalty for the sins of those who would put their trust in Him. Thus we have access to the throne of grace from which all blessings come. As one historic prayer of consecration puts it: ". . . Through faith in His blood, we and all Thy whole Church have remission of our sins *and all other benefits of His passion*" (*Book of Common Prayer*, p. 335, italics added). Those who make Jesus Christ their Lord and Savior, in other words, are offered healing for their spiritual sickness and other blessings as well, including physical and emotional healing.

2. The Communion elements are consecrated to be the body and blood of Christ and to be vehicles for the mediation of grace. Many Christians, especially those of certain Protestant backgrounds, have trouble with the idea that the Communion elements are means of bestowing God's grace, until they recall a basic truth: God uses material things to flesh out spiritual reality. One man asked me once, "How could God bestow blessing through a piece of bread and a sip of wine after certain words were said over them?" I asked him if he had any difficulty in accepting the truth that the second Person of the Godhead lived on earth as a human being with flesh, blood and bones. He got the point. The God who took flesh also uses material objects as some of the ways He comes to us and bestows blessings.

Just as Jesus is not a *symbol* for God, but is literally God made flesh, so too do the Communion elements do more than just *symbolize* spiritual reality. They *are* spiritual reality—the body and blood of Jesus—and they convey spiritual blessing. I have known people healed of various physical, emotional and spiritual ailments as they took holy Communion. Many of them were not even thinking about their need for healing as they received the elements.

Healing Ministry with a Prayer Team

Although this is not part of the Eucharistic liturgy as such, a growing number of churches have teams of lay people available in a side chapel, or in a corner of the main church, to pray for people right after they receive Communion. With the reminder of what Christ did for them at Calvary fresh in their minds, and with His body and blood just consumed, they are ready to meet God in a focused, intentional prayer for healing.

Closing Prayers and Dismissal

In the closing prayer we thank God for what He has done for us—whether in visible manifestations of His grace, in ways we will not discover until later or in general ways of blessing us—and we ask Him to strengthen us for service in His name. One prayer often used contains these words: ". . . Send us out to do the work You have given us to do. . . ." Part of that work is to minister healing through leading people to salvation in Christ (*always* the most important healing a person can receive), by praying for or with people to be healed and by working for the healing of society.

The words of dismissal—"Let us go forth in the name of Christ" or "Go in peace to love and serve the Lord" or "Let us go forth into the world, rejoicing in the power of the Spirit," etc.—give us our marching orders and the name under which we minister. I knew one priest who occasionally used to say at the dismissal, "Go get 'em, Christians!"

As we understand the tremendous healing power of the Eucharist and that every Communion service is a healing service, we will want to receive Communion more often. And as we understand that Communion was the service observed every Sunday by the Church since the days of the apostles, we may even join the ranks of the many who are demanding that every Sunday service be a service of Communion.

May Christians Judge?

May Christians stand in judgment? Christians are constantly being told, "Don't be judgmental." The text cited is Matthew 7:1–2: "Judge not, that you be not judged. For with the judgment you pronounce you will be judged, and the measure you give will be the measure you get."

We recognize that the judgmental attitudes we all slip into are not in keeping with Christian love. But aren't there times when we simply have to judge? We would not leave our children with just any babysitter. We would find out whether or not he or she was competent, reliable and mature. Nor would we blindly accept any teaching that comes along but would test it to see if it is from God (1 John 4:1).

There are times when we have to make judgments. Far from forbidding us to do this, the Bible even exhorts us to judge: "Do you not know that the saints [that is, God's people] will judge the world? . . . Do you not know that we are to judge angels? How much more, matters pertaining to this life!" (1 Corinthians 6:2–3). Scripture cannot contradict itself because it is God-breathed (the literal meaning of the word *theopneustos*, usually translated "inspired") and God is not self-contradictory. How then do we reconcile these seemingly conflicting statements?

The Greek of the New Testament makes it clear that two different types of judgment are meant. The judgment that is wrong—the judgment that Matthew 7:1–2 rules out—uses the Greek word *krino*. It means to pass judgment on, to decide, conclude, condemn. The judgment that is right uses several other Greek words—*dokimazo, anakrino, diakrino*. The meaning is to test, investigate, search out, weigh, examine or discern. There are a number of ways we can test ourselves to see if an attitude or action is judgmental (wrong) or discerning (right).

1. Judgment forms opinions on first impressions, on hearsay or on secondary evidence. Discernment withholds forming an opinion until it checks things for accuracy and does it firsthand with the person involved.

Judgment is quick to believe something because it appeared that way on the surface, or because someone else said it was so. Discernment goes to the person directly and seeks clarification. How many times have I passed judgment on the basis of what someone told me, only to discover that things were not as they had been related to me? It was not that people had necessarily been lying to me. We hear and see selectively and we inadvertently garble things when we tell others. Jesus' message in the Temple needs to be grafted onto our hearts: "Do not judge by appearances, but judge with right judgment" (John 7:24).

2. Judgment condemns others without getting oneself in order. Discernment examines self first before presuming to go to others.

It is often the case that those sins we hate in others are our own worst faults! Paul told the Romans that "in passing judgment upon [others] you condemn yourself, because you, the judge, are doing the very same things" (Romans 2:1). Jesus tells us in the Sermon on the Mount that we should first take the log out of our own eye so that we can see clearly to take the speck out of our brother's (Matthew 7:3–5). Note that both the logs and the specks are made of the same substance—wood. Jesus' statement does not mean we are not to point out to other people their faults. Rather, He says we can come to a position where we can see clearly enough to remove other people's specks. What He means is for us to get our own spiritual house generally in order first. As a result, when we go to others it will be with the humility of one who has "been there." On such occasions we will have love in our "tough love."

3. Judgment has as its purpose destruction. Discernment has as its purpose restoration.

From time to time Christians, especially those in leadership positions, are called on to deliver a sharp, strong, prophetic message to someone. Paul told Titus to watch out for those dwellers of Crete over whom Paul had appointed him bishop. In strong language Paul referred to them as "liars, evil beasts, lazy gluttons" (Titus 1:12). Titus was told to rebuke them sharply. The difference between judgment and discernment is not always sharp rebuke versus tender words. The difference has to do with motive. Titus was told to rebuke them not in order to tear them down, but so "that they may be sound in the faith" (verse 13).

Before you go to other people to point out their faults, ask yourself why you are going. Is it to tear them down or to build them up? It is usually easy to distinguish the two in ourselves. When we tear down, we glare, use harsh words, speak with an attitude of putting the other persons down, are little interested in what they have to say. Our emotions are out of control. When we go to build up, we choose our words more carefully, have the desire to see the others do well, sometimes even have tears in our eyes. Usually, though not always, we speak in a moderate tone and are in control of ourselves.

Since we cannot always gauge accurately whether our motive is destruction or restoration, it may be helpful to check it out with someone who will be honest with us.

4. Judgment condemns the person involved. Discernment condemns the action but loves the person.

One day when Jesus was teaching in the Temple, He was brought a woman who had been caught in the act of adultery (John 8:1–11). He was asked, "What do you say about her?" He was being presented with the opportunity to be either judging or discerning. In saying, "Go and do not sin again," Jesus made it clear that her actions were out of the will of God. Yet He, God's Son, who of anyone on earth had the right to be judgmental, refused to condemn the woman.

Before we go to other people to point out their faults, we need to make sure of two things. *First, we must make sure that their actions are actually sins according to Scripture.* On the one hand we may gloss over or excuse things that the Bible condemns. In that case we may tolerate or even applaud behavior that God wants stopped.

When we do this we are not being loving to others. We are failing to sound a needed, though unpleasant, warning. On the other hand we may deem as sin something that is merely a difference in personality or culture. In that case we may condemn an action that is not against God's will.

Second, we must take care to distinguish between condemning persons and condemning sin. If you are having a difficult time doing this, take some time to reflect on how you appreciate being loved by those who talk to you about your sins. In addition, take some time to pray—lovingly, positively—for the person you are going to confront.

5. Judgment deals with matters publicly. It gossips and seeks to make others judge the person. Discernment deals with the matter privately. It goes to the person directly and involves no one else, until bringing in others is appropriate.

Often our judgment against a person causes us to tell others our feelings, hoping they will side with us in our judgment. Jesus carefully outlined the procedure we must follow when we act on what we perceive are the sins of others. In Matthew 18:15 He said, "If your brother sins against you, go and tell him his fault, *between you and him alone"* (italics added). If he refuses to hear, the next verse tells us to involve one or two others, so long as they are people who are *already* involved ("the evidence of two or three witnesses"). We are not to go get people who were not present at or involved in the particular offense, tell them our version of the story and get them to take up our cause with us.

Even if we are able to withstand the obvious temptation to line up otherwise uninvolved people, we must guard against the more subtle temptation to phrase our gossip as a "prayer request": "Please pray for John. He's in need of God's help because of his sin of. . . ."

6. Judgment is nosy. It butts in where it has no business, and speaks at times and in ways the Lord has not led. Discernment is needful. It is involved only when it has the right to be, and when and how the Lord directs.

Often we get hot and steamy, come to false conclusions and involve ourselves in things that are none of our business. It is not always up to us to take up another person's cause and get angry for them. It is often our job to help others deal with their problems in the proper way. People with spiritual discernment know, moreover, that some revelations are for keeping, not for sharing. That is to say, on some occasions we are allowed to recognize the faults of others, not to go to them but to hold them before God in prayer.

A Final Note

Why is it so important that we distinguish between judging and discerning?

1. Because we all need help getting rid of occasional judgmental thoughts or deeds. By familiarizing ourselves with what constitutes being judgmental, we will better be able to identify such actions and attitudes and, with the Lord's help, take corrective action.

2. So we will not go to the opposite extreme. Many people who will not take a stand on anything, or who cannot assert scriptural truth with conviction, act that way because formerly they were judgmental. But one extreme is just as bad as the other. To be able to avoid being judgmental can help us from swinging to the opposite error.

3. To protect the biblical ministry of building up one another into maturity. Often our discerning words to other people strike raw nerves in them. They do not want to deal with their sins so they attack the person who brought them a discerning word as being judgmental, harsh, critical, unloving. In other words, "If you don't like the message, attack the messenger" with whatever is handy. For many, what is handy is a misuse of the word *judgmental*.

Often the effect on those bringing discerning correctives is devastating. They do not want to be judgmental and they certainly do not want to be yelled at. Thus, they reason, maybe they had better stop saying anything. This is detrimental to the Church because it means there will be little or no building up one another into maturity, no nipping sin in the bud. After a while we become a church of wimps and Satan wins a victory.

In this time of great theological and moral crisis in churches, it is crucial that we know we are doing God's will when we take biblical stands in appropriate ways. God's truth done in God's love is what is needed now.

Case Study
Review Questions

We should be careful to remember that no matter how tired we are, or how distracted by our own cares, or how many people to whom we have ministered on a particular day or through the years, each person deserves our best. One way to keep this in mind is to remember that every person to whom we minister is precious to God and should be precious to us. In addition, each time we minister to someone we are presented with a situation that can be reviewed and discussed (but only in an appropriate manner) with our prayer partners and with those supervising us.

We find that Jesus trained His disciples and sent them out (Matthew 10:1ff). Nevertheless, they did not get it right all the time and needed their ministries reviewed (Matthew 17:14–21). Similarly, from time to time it is helpful for us to review our ministries by selecting an occasion of ministry to a person and making it a "case study." The purpose is to review occasions of ministry to see if we made some mistakes that need to be rectified, to learn how we can do better the next time and to identify what spiritual and personal issues have come to the surface. Far from depersonalizing those to whom we minister, such case studies help us to be even more helpful to them. Here are several points to ponder in your review.

Practical

1. Did the person to whom you were ministering cry when you prayed? Did you have facial tissues handy?

2. Was he or she overcome by the Spirit? Were there trained "catchers" ready? Did you have something handy with which to cover those lying in a way that would have embarrassed them?

3. Was the deployment of the teams such that there was sufficient privacy for prayer?

4. Did you encounter a "problem person" (for example, someone who tried to tell you his life story when only a brief description of the immediate problem was appropriate, or who insisted you pray longer than the appropriate amount of time)? How did you handle the situation? On further reflection, how will you handle it in the future?

5. Was there someone who so lost composure as to embarrass himself or significantly disturb others? How should this situation be handled?

6. If you sensed there were various gifts of the Spirit (such as prophecy, a word of knowledge or a word of wisdom) to be manifested, what did you do? Were there practical problems in using them? Did the people for whom you prayed seem comfortable with the manifestations of the Spirit?

7. Were there logistical problems in praying together with others on your prayer team? Was there someone clearly in charge? Did he or she know what to do and do it confidently, yet gently? Did each person on the team know his or her role and yet have sufficient freedom to minister as the Spirit led?

8. Did you have enough time with each person or did you feel rushed? What could be done about this?

9. Did people who wanted prayer need to stand while waiting their turn?

10. How did people who could not get to the altar for prayer signal their needs so that a healing team could go to them in their pew?

11. Was the prayer team physically comfortable during the prayer session? If not, how could the situation be altered?

Theological and Spiritual

1. Were theological questions raised by the people to whom you were ministering, questions for which you did not have a biblically sound, brief answer? What were those questions and what are you doing to find out the answers?
2. What theological questions arose in you?
3. Are you actively seeking the gifts of the Spirit? Do you sense God starting to use you in various of the spiritual gifts? What have you experienced so far? What are you doing to make sure you are staying theologically sound in your understanding of them? What are you doing to make sure you are staying balanced in your use of them?
4. Did you find your confrontation with human pain and misery affecting your relationship with God? In what way? If negatively, what are you doing about it?
5. Because of your ministering healing, have you noticed increased temptation or the experience of those "little nastinesses" Satan throws at those trying to roll back his rule? How can you prepare better spiritually for next time?
6. Have you added to or altered your prayer practice because of your experiences in ministering?
7. Did you sense the move of the Spirit in you? In the others on the team?

Psychological

1. Were you "appropriately compassionate"? (Or were you too emotionally caught up with the problems of the people to whom you ministered? Were you too detached?)
2. Did the needs of a particular person or persons remind you of loved ones who had suffered similarly? Were you aware of your emotional response to the remembrances during the time of ministry?
3. Did they remind you of needs or hurts you have experienced personally?
4. Did they remind you of painful things you had repressed from conscious thought?

5. Were you aware of "projection"—that is, saying or doing things that are directed more appropriately toward yourself than to others?
6. Were you aware of the emotional issues of your own future illness and death?
7. Did you feel discouraged about people returning for prayer over unresolved issues or problems? How did you handle it?

Notes

Chapter One

1. The Lausanne Committee for Evangelism, a distinguished international group representing the evangelical Protestant segment of the Church, commented recently on the place of healing in the life of the Church: "Jesus did more than preach the kingdom; he demonstrated its reality with 'signs of the kingdom,' public evidence that the kingdom he was talking about had come. We believe that signs should validate our evangelism, too. . ." (*Evangelism and Social Responsibility*, Lausanne Occasional Paper No. 21 [Grand Rapids: 1982], pp. 31–32). This statement is significant coming from a wing of the Church not usually friendly to the ministry of healing.

Chapter Four

1. This example comes from Oscar Cullman in his book *Christ & Time.*

2. See Appendix 6 for a few case studies demonstrating this.

Chapter Five

1. But as examples of sickness as punishment, please note how the Lord sent a plague on the people because they made the golden calf (Exodus 32:35); how He promises to make sick the false

prophetess Jezebel and strike dead her children for encouraging people to commit fornication (Revelation 2:20–23); and the dire consequences of partaking of the Lord's Supper in an unworthy manner (1 Corinthians 11:27–30). On occasion God may do such a thing; He has every right to. On other occasions God may send sickness for the greater good of getting our attention so that we will turn to Him in repentance and faith. Paul's temporary blindness on the road to Damascus (Acts 9:8–9) is an example of this.

2. For a more in-depth treatment of how Christians may appropriately bring tough love confrontation to those in sin, see Appendix 8, "May Christians Judge?"

3. For a helpful book on how church discipline, done correctly, is a great blessing to God's people, see John White and Ken Blue, *Healing the Wounded: The Costly Love of Church Discipline,* published by InterVarsity Press.

Chapter Eight

1. For a good understanding of how spiritual renewal must be grounded in personal reform, see *The Reform of Renewal* by Benedict J. Groeschel, C.F.R. (Ignatius Press, 1990).

Chapter Nine

1. I demonstrate the way different personality types often prefer different styles of worship, Bible study, prayer and Christian service in my book *Why Can't I Be Me?* (Chosen Books, 1992). See especially chapter 7.

2. For a fuller treatment of the various aspects of how the service of Communion can work for healing, see Appendix 7, pages 328–334. For a book-length treatment, see *Healing through the Mass* by the Rev. Robert De Grandis, SSJ (Resurrection Press, 1992). Although Roman Catholic in orientation, there is little in the book that would not apply equally to people of nearly all Christian groups.

3. The book is entitled *Christian Initiation and Baptism in the Holy Spirit: Evidence from the First Eight Centuries* (Collegeville, Minn.: The Liturgical Press, 1991). A brief summary is the minibook *Fanning the Flame,* same publisher and date.

Chapter Eleven

1. It is quite possible for a person to assent to particular Christian truths while having a basically secular worldview. For a discerning presentation of the importance of a consistently Christian worldview, see *The Christian Mind: How Should a Christian Think?* by Harry Blamires (Servant Books, Ann Arbor, 1978). Blamires' tutor at Oxford was C. S. Lewis, some of whose brilliance rubbed off onto his pupil.

Chapter Twelve

1. A classic example is *Interior Castle* by St. Teresa of Avila. *The Spiritual Exercises of St. Ignatius* is ideal for the study of discerning God's guidance through the movement of the heart and mind in prayer. Thomas Green's *Weeds Among the Wheat* is an excellent modern counterpart. A modern-day mystic, Carlo Carretto, provides a "little course" in understanding mystical encounter and guidance in all of his books, but perhaps especially in *Why, O Lord?*, *Blessed Are You Who Believed* and *The God Who Comes*.

Chapter Thirteen

1. Those offering ministry need to discuss the progress of the ministry from time to time with their supervisor. A good rule of thumb is to evaluate after five or six sessions before deciding to continue. If little progress is being made, one needs to ask why. Sometimes it is because we are not gifted in the area needing attention. Sometimes it is because a specially trained, professional counselor is needed. Sometimes it is because our original diagnosis was incorrect. We also have to be aware that our need to be needed can so get in the way that we get people dependent on us and ask them to keep coming back.

Chapter Fourteen

1. See *Why Can't I Be Me?* by Mark A. Pearson for a thorough discussion of how different personality types communicate differently.

Recommended Reading

The last fifteen years have seen an explosion of good books on Christian healing. What follows is but a brief summary of some of these.

Introductory, Overview Books

Healing by Dr. Francis MacNutt. Ave Maria Press.

The Power to Heal by Dr. Francis MacNutt. Discussion of such issues as "soaking prayer," suffering and death, being "slain in the Spirit," faith vs. presumption. Ave Maria Press.

The Healings of Jesus by the Rev. Canon Michael Harper. A careful examination of each of the New Testament accounts of our Lord's healing work. Excellent for Bible study purposes. Inter-Varsity Press.

Your Healing Is Within You by the Rev. Canon James Glennon. James Glennon is one of the leaders in Christian healing in Australia. Bridge Publishing, Inc.

Trinity of Man by the Rev. Canon Dennis J. and Rita Bennett. Healing the whole person—spirit, soul and body. New Leaf Press.

Healing: God's Work Among Us by the Rev. John Bertolucci. Answers to such questions as, Why do we, as disciples of Jesus, sometimes experience pain, sickness and suffering? Fr. John is America's best-known Roman Catholic evangelist. Servant Publications.

The Adventures of Healing by the Rev. Dr. Donald W. Bartow. A helpful resource workbook that provides needed references, capsule summaries, quick overviews and scriptural citations by a man who, for many years, has been a leader in Christian healing in the Presbyterian Church. Life Enrichment Publishers.

Authority to Heal by Ken Blue. An introductory volume on the authority and practice of healing. InterVarsity Press.

Celebration of Healing by Emily Gardiner Neal. A posthumous collection from the various writings of this pioneer in the healing ministry. Her initial book, *A Reporter Finds God through Spiritual Healing*, first published in 1956, went through fifteen printings and significantly helped the revival of the healing ministry in our day. Cowley Publications.

The Gospel of Healing by A. B. Simpson. Simpson was a significant figure in Christian history and was founder of the Christian and Missionary Alliance denomination. He wrote this book more than a hundred years ago, long before the present healing movement began. Christian Publications.

Healing in Church History

Psychology, Medicine and Christian Healing by the Rev. Dr. Morton T. Kelsey. The author, an Episcopal priest and long-time professor at the University of Notre Dame, gives a thorough examination of healing in the first centuries of the life of the Church. There is also a lengthy study of the interrelationship of the body and emotions according to Jungian psychology. HarperCollins.

Biblical Healing: Hebrew and Christian Roots by Professor Frank C. Darling. A "primary source texts" reader with biblical and patristic quotes. Author is a retired political scientist and a practicing Christian Scientist. Vista Publications, P.O. Box 302, Boulder, CO 80306.

Christian Healing in the Middle Ages and Beyond by Professor Frank C. Darling. Vista Publications.

The Restoration of Christian Healing: New Freedom in the Church Since the Reformation by Professor Frank C. Darling. A thorough church historical analysis of movements of and important persons in healing since 1500. Emphasis is placed on the Reformation, on post-Reformation revival movements, on meta-physical/New Thought groups and on twentieth-century leaders. Vista Publications.

The Healing of Memories/Inner Healing

Five Loaves and Two Fishes by Phoebe Cranor. Practical assistance for those seeking inner healing to locate the painful areas of their pasts, offer them to Jesus and experience transformation. Paulist Press.

Healing for Damaged Emotions by the Rev. Dr. David A. Seamands. A veteran Methodist pastor and seminary professor shares his insights on the healings of a variety of emotional difficulties. Scripture Press Publishers, Inc.

My Father's Child—Help and Healing for the Victims of Emotional, Sexual, and Physical Abuse by Lynda D. Elliott and Dr. Vicki L. Tanner. The authors are Christian counselors. Wolgemuth & Hyatt, Publishers, Inc.

Biblical Inner Healing by the Rev. Dr. F. Earle Fox. An explanation of the biblical roots of the healing of memories, a biblical understanding of the unconscious and other foundation stones for a biblically based psychology. Emmaus Ministries, 718 Maplewood Ave., Ambridge, PA 15003.

Healing the Hidden Self by Barbara Shlemon (Ryan), R.N. Six major stages of development—conception and life in the womb, birth, infancy, childhood, adolescence, young adulthood and adulthood—are discussed, showing how emotional hurt and damage to the inner self is possible, damage that may not manifest until much later. Practical, useful help toward setting people free. Ave Maria Press.

The Transformation of the Inner Man by the Rev. John and Paula Sandford. The most comprehensive book on inner healing in print. Victory House, Inc.

A Comprehensive Guide to Deliverance and Inner Healing by John and Mark Sandford. Stresses the interdependence of deliverance and inner healing, showing how both are valuable and necessary. Chosen Books.

The Healing Presence by Leanne Payne. Practical guidance to help hurting people open their hearts to gain access to Christ's healing presence. An honest account of the possibilities and problems in gaining "victorious Christian living." Crossway Books.

Healing of Memories by the Rev. Dr. David A. Seamands. How God's healing power can free people from the tyranny of painful memories that affect behavior and Christian growth. Victor Books.

Why Can't I Be Me? by the Rev. Canon Mark A. Pearson. Sometimes emotional wounding occurs at the hands of otherwise loving and caring parents, teachers and clergy, if they try to force an individual to adopt a different personality from the one God gave. This book applies the Myers-Briggs Type Indicator to inner healing, interpersonal relationships, working together in a team setting and the spiritual life. Chosen Books.

Healing the Wounds of Divorce by Barbara Shlemon (Ryan), R.N. Seventeen short chapters dealing with practical issues such as children, finances and relatives, and spiritual concerns such as fear, guilt and forgiveness. Ave Maria Press.

Love Is a Choice: Recovery for Codependent Relationships by Drs. Robert Hemfelt, Frank Minirth and Paul Meier. A balanced, helpful, biblically sound treatment of the problem of codependency, with suggestions toward healing. Thomas Nelson Publishers.

Twelve Steps for Christians by several anonymous Christians. Each of the steps of the classic Twelve Step programs (such as Alcoholics Anonymous) applied to various addictions and dysfunctions. Lots of Scripture references. Recovery Publications.

A Hunger for Healing by J. Keith Miller. The Twelve Steps as a model for wholeness. HarperCollins.

Restoring the Christian Soul through Healing Prayer by Leanne Payne. Three great barriers, according to the author, keep individuals from becoming whole—inability to receive God's forgiveness, inability to forgive others and inability to accept ourselves. How to overcome these and become free. Crossway Books.

Healing the Wounded Spirit by the Rev. John and Paula Sandford. Chapters on a whole variety of things that can hurt emotionally, such as anorexia, rejection, depression, frustration. Chapters on problems in the womb and intergenerational problems. Victory House, Inc.

Healing Victims of Sexual Abuse by Paula Sandford. Love, acceptance and healing to all the victims—the abused, the abuser and their families. A valuable tool for those who minister. Victory House, Inc.

Making Peace with Your Inner Child by Rita Bennett. Dealing with the conscious and subconscious record of the emotions, hurts and bad experiences of the childhood years. Fleming H. Revell Co.

Sexuality and the Healing of Sexual Identity Disorders

The Broken Image by Leanne Payne. Steps to healing for those with various sexual identity crises. The author is both a scholar on the writings of C. S. Lewis and one who has had a successful ministry to those with sexuality disorders. Good News Publishers.

Crisis in Masculinity by Leanne Payne. What does it mean to be male, and how can men affirm that God-given heritage without reverting to wimpiness or overreacting to being macho? Good News Publishers.

Steps Out of Homosexuality by Frank Worthen. A compassionate book written by a man whose ministry to men and women overcoming homosexuality is worldwide. Love in Action, Inc.

You Don't Have to Be Gay by ex-gay J. A. Konrad. A nontechnical book for those who desire to understand homosexuality and its root causes. Conversationally written as a series of letters to a despondent young man unfulfilled in his homosexuality. Pacific Publishing House.

The Courage to Be Chaste by the Rev. Benedict J. Groeschel, C.F.R. Helpful guidance to those who are unmarried. Paulist Press.

Healing the Masculine Soul by the Rev. Gordon Dalbey. The author is a United Church of Christ pastor who twice won the Billings prize in preaching at Harvard University and served in the Peace Corps. Word, Inc.

Counseling the Homosexual by Michael Saia. Thorough and well-balanced. Bethany House Publishers.

Biblical Sexuality and the Battle for Science by the Rev. Dr. F. Earle Fox. Discussion of various issues facing the Church today: the "new morality," homosexual unions, the failure of Kinseyan sexology and more. The author has an earned doctorate from Oxford in the theology and philosophy of science. Emmaus Ministries, 718 Maplewood Ave., Ambridge, PA 15003.

Human Sexuality: Hetero-, Homo-, or Pan-? by the Rev. Dr. F. Earle Fox. Emmaus Ministries.

Unnatural Affections: The Impuritan Ethic of Homosexuality and the Modern Church by George Grant and Mark Horne. A response to the insurgent forces in the mainline churches favoring homosexual practice. Legacy Press, Box 680365, Franklin, TN 37068.

Evil, Demons, Satan, Deliverance and Exorcism

Spiritual Warfare by the Rev. Canon Michael Harper. Basic overview of the subject of evil in the world, and the context for study about and combat against the demonic. Servant Publications.

The Screwtape Letters by C. S. Lewis. A humorous account of the subject as told from the demons' side. Long a classic. In several editions.

Deliverance from Evil Spirits by the Rev. Michael Scanlan, T.O.R. A basic manual for deliverance from evil spirits by a Roman Catholic priest/university president. Servant Publications.

Demon Possession edited by Dr. John Warwick Montgomery. The papers of a medical, historical, anthropological and theological symposium held under the auspices of the Christian Medical Association. The most comprehensive, scholarly book on the subject. Bethany House Publishers.

The Beautiful Side of Evil by Johanna Michaelsen. The story of a young woman who, while in search of spiritual truth, became involved in occultic healing. She tells from firsthand experience how some healings can come from evil spiritual powers, which initially masquerade as beneficial and godly. Harvest House Publishers.

This Present Darkness and *Piercing the Darkness* by Frank E. Peretti. Two runaway bestselling novels highlighting the dangers of New Age occultism. Good News Publishers.

Demon Possession & the Christian by C. Fred Dickason. A thorough, well-referenced book. Theologically sound, practical. Crossway Books.

Exposing the Prince of Darkness by the Rev. Canon Michael Green. Theological treatment of spiritual warfare, recognizing satanic strategies, understanding demonization, discernment and deliverance, wielding authority as a believer. Vine Books/Servant Publications.

Deliver Us from Evil by the Rev. Don Basham. Firsthand accounts of a latter-day pioneer in the deliverance ministry. Chosen Books.

Satan Stalking by Dorothy Marie England (pseudonym). Firsthand account of a woman's encounter with evil spirits. Forward Movement Publications.

Defeating Dark Angels: Breaking Demonic Oppression in the Believer's Life by Charles H. Kraft. How demons operate and how to take authority over them. Solid but readable text by a professor at Fuller Theological Seminary. Servant Publications.

Overcoming the Dominion of Darkness: Personal Strategies for Spiritual Warfare by Gary D. Kinnaman. Resource for recognizing, resisting and overcoming the powers of Satan. Chosen Books.

The New Age Movement

Unmasking the New Age by Douglas R. Groothuis. A basic overview of the sources, beliefs and dangers. InterVarsity Press.

Confronting the New Age by Douglas R. Groothuis. New Age views as expressed in business sales seminars, educational curriculum, pop psychology, visualization techniques and music. The author refrains from legalistic condemnations and guilt by association, but rather sorts out what is good from what is not in these areas. InterVarsity Press.

Revealing the New Age Jesus by Douglas R. Groothuis. A comparison between Orthodox Christian and New Age beliefs about Jesus. InterVarsity Press.

Reincarnation by Mark C. Albrecht. A basic overview and Christian response, from Scripture and the writings of the early Church. Answers to the seeming evidence for past-life recall. Philosophical and moral objections to reincarnation. InterVarsity Press.

Christian Science by Dr. Walter R. Martin. An examination and critique of its teachings. Bethany House Publishers.

Shirley MacLaine and the New Age Movement by James W. Sire. A quick overview of New Age beliefs as made popular by their best-known spokesperson, with Christian answers. InterVarsity Press.

Reincarnation and Christianity: Has the Traditional Viewpoint of the Church Been Right? by Robert A. Morey. Bethany House Publishers.

When the New Age Gets Old by Vishal Mangalwadi. A thorough examination of various New Age beliefs and practices written by a native of India. The author experienced and studied various beliefs and practices of the New Age Movement firsthand. InterVarsity Press.

Evangelizing the New Age by Paul McGuire. How Christians can reclaim "territory" and people for the Lord from the New Age Movement. Vine Books/Servant Publications.

Scripture Twisting by James Sire. Various ways cults misinterpret the Bible for their own ends. Good for understanding how the New Age Movement uses Scripture but in different ways from orthodox Christianity. InterVarsity Press.

The Universe Next Door by James Sire. Chapters on various Eastern religions. InterVarsity Press.

The Holistic Healers by Paul C. Reisser, Teri K. Reisser and John Weldon. InterVarsity Press.

Psychology as Religion by Paul Vitz. Critiques of various influential psychologists and their philosophies. Eerdmans.

Jesus: Ghost, God, or Guru? by Jon Buell and O. Quentin Hyder. Brief, convincing argument for the unique deity of Christ. Zondervan.

The Authentic Jesus by the Rev. Dr. John R. W. Stott. Defends biblical view of Jesus. InterVarsity Press.

Knowing the Truth about the Resurrection by William L. Craig. An easy-to-read defense of the resurrection of Jesus. Servant Publications.

Speaking the Christian God: The Holy Trinity and the Challenge of Feminism edited by the Rev. Alvin F. Kimel, Jr. A comprehensive critique of radical feminism's radical reconceptualization of Christian theology. By a variety of authors. Eerdmans.

The Cruelty of Heresy by the Rt. Rev. C. FitzSimons Allison. Explores the historical roots of persistent heresies of the Christian faith; profiles great defenders of the faith; and examines the fallacies of popular contemporary heresies.

The Sacraments

To Heal as Jesus Healed by Barbara Shlemon (Ryan), R.N., and the Revs. Matthew and Dennis Linn. A discussion of the relationship between healing prayer and the sacrament of unction (anointing the sick). Bringing together the present-day experience of the Holy Spirit's power and the ancient liturgical rites of the Church, the authors show how they naturally belong together and need each other. They illustrate with moving personal examples how any crippling illness is an opportunity for emotional, spiritual and especially physical healing. Ave Maria Press.

And Their Eyes Were Opened—Encountering Jesus in the Sacraments by the Rev. Michael Scanlan, T.O.R., and Sister Ann Therese Shields. While written only in part about healing, an excellent book to help those in liturgical churches unite personal piety and sacramental participation. Servant Publications.

Healing through the Mass by the Rev. Robert DeGrandis, S.J. The author walks the reader through each step of the Eucharist, demonstrating how it can be a healing service. While written in a Roman Catholic context, Christians from other churches can find innumerable valuable insights. Resurrection Press.

The Power in Penance by the Rev. Michael Scanlan, T.O.R. James 5:16 tells us to confess our sins to one another. This little book describes how this may be done in a sacramental context. Ave Maria Press.

Miracles Do Happen by Sister Briege McKenna, O.S.C. Healings associated with faithful participation in the Eucharist. Veritas Publications.

Spiritual Gifts

Your Spiritual Gifts Can Help Your Church Grow by Dr. C. Peter Wagner. A thorough discussion of each of the spiritual gifts and how they can be used harmoniously for the glory of God and the betterment of God's people. Regal Books.

Spiritual Gifts in the Local Church—How to Integrate Them into the Ministry of the People of God by the Rt. Rev. David Pytches. The author, for many years an Anglican bishop in South America, examines the various spiritual gifts and gives wise advice on how they can be used sanely in local churches. Bethany House Publishers.

Discovering Your Spiritual Gifts by the Rev. Kenneth C. Kinghorn. Brief introduction to the subject written with the average layperson in mind. Abingdon.

Overcome by the Spirit by Dr. Francis MacNutt. The phenomenon of being overcome by the Spirit (sometimes called being "slain in the Spirit") is neither new, nor American, nor particularly Pentecostal. This short book gives a theological and historical background, as well as guidance on how to discern a genuine experience from a spurious one. Chosen Books.

Fire in the Fireplace by Dr. Charles E. Hummel. One of the great classic books in the charismatic renewal, now issued in a revised and expanded edition. A careful description and evaluation of the various aspects of the current renewal movement. The title illustrates the author's purpose—to put the fire of renewal into the fireplace of biblical scholarship, historical context, careful discernment, orderly expression and the like. InterVarsity Press.

I Believe in the Holy Spirit by the Rev. Canon Michael Green. An in-depth theological treatment by a long-respected English evangelical Anglican. Besides advocating participation in the full life of the Spirit, the author offers wise guidance and sounds appropriate warnings. Eerdmans.

The Gifts of the Spirit by Judith MacNutt, Jack Hayford, Michael P. Williams, Mark A. Pearson, John Archer, Mahesh Chavda, Reinhardt Bonnke and John Wimber. A mini-book overview. Creation House.

Christian Initiation and Baptism in the Holy Spirit by the Revs. Kilian McDonnell, O.S.B., and George Montague, S.M. Early post-biblical and patristic evidence for the baptism in the Holy Spirit as normative and integral to Christian initiation and discipleship. The Liturgical Press.

Fanning the Flame by the same authors. A much briefer version of the above book. The Liturgical Press.

Prophecy in the Church by Martin Scott. Brief mini-book introduction to the theology and practice of the gift of prophecy. Creation House.

Miracles Never Cease! by Oral Roberts, William DeArteaga, Paul Thigpen and Jack Deere. Mini-book treatment of such questions about the miraculous as, Did the power of the Spirit ever leave the Church? Why does God perform miracles? Why don't we see as many as the New Testament Church did? Creation House.

Christianity with Power by Charles H. Kraft. An evangelical moves past his previously limited understanding of the miraculous to discover the importance of present-day, supernatural, divine power. Vine Books of Servant Publications.

The Collapse of the Brass Heaven: Rebuilding Our Worldview to Embrace the Power of God by the Rev. Dr. Zeb Bradford Long and the Rev. Douglas McMurry. How the Western Church has become separated from the spiritual world, and a call back to biblical faith in the power of God. Chosen Books.

Having a Healing Ministry in Your Church

Healing Prayer by Barbara Shlemon (Ryan), R.N. A practical guide to praying for the sick by a registered nurse who was also instrumental in forming the Association of Christian Therapists. Ave Maria Press.

Blessed to Be a Blessing—How to Have an Intentional Healing Ministry in Your Church by the Rev. Dr. James K. Wagner. Many practical suggestions by a United Methodist minister who introduced the healing ministry into the several churches he pastored. Upper Room Books.

How to Have a Healing Ministry in Any Church by Dr. C. Peter Wagner. The author, a professor at Fuller Theological Seminary, gives practical suggestions on how to introduce a healing ministry to a church without either splitting it or turning it Pentecostal. Regal Books.

The Heart of a Healthy Body—Helping People Find Healing and Wholeness through the Body of Christ by the Rev. Dr. Herbert

Beuoy. The author successfully introduced the ministry of healing into two mainline United Methodist churches, overcoming
his and their skepticism. Upper Room Books.

An Adventure in Healing & Wholeness by the Rev. Dr. James K.
Wagner. A seven-session, self-guided workbook version of the
author's workshop on healing and wholeness. Upper Room
Books.

The Wounded Healer by the Rev. Henri J. M. Nouwen. Long a classic, this book offers guidance to those who would minister to
others. Doubleday.

Channels of Healing Prayer by the Rev. Benedict Heron, O.S.B.
Helpful suggestions on how people can pray for others. Ave
Maria Press.

Other Books About Healing

Fear No Evil by the Rev. Canon David C. K. Watson. This book
by a leader in the renewal in England is his diary of reflections,
hopes, fears and experiences of God in his last few years on earth
before his premature death. It is a reminder that even those who
have broad understanding and an experience of spiritual healing for others may have difficulty receiving it for themselves, but
that God is always faithful. Harold Shaw Press.

Praying for Your Unborn Child by Dr. Francis and Judith MacNutt.
Write the authors: "We believe that, if enough parents start praying for their unborn children . . . the babies to be born will
become a new, different generation—more disposed to love
God, happier and more secure." Doubleday.

The Compulsive Woman by Sandra Simpson LeSourd. How to break
the bonds of addiction to food, television, sex, men, exercise,
shopping, alcohol, drugs, nicotine and much more. Chosen
Books.

The Not-So-Compulsive Woman by Sandra Simpson LeSourd.
Twenty recovery principles for enjoying freedom from people-
pleasing, male dependency, perfectionism, etc. Chosen Books.

Whatever Became of Sin? by Dr. Karl Menninger. A psychiatrist from
the famed Menninger Clinic urges the clergy to affirm their
unique calling and to preach comfort, repentance, hope,
acknowledgment and forgiveness of sin. Hawthorne Books, Inc.

The Healing of Persons by Dr. Paul Tournier. A renowned Swiss physician views the patient as a body-soul-spirit whole person, and relates physical health to healing of the soul and spirit. A classic and noteworthy contribution to the growth in understanding of whole-person medicine. HarperCollins.

Good Grief by Dr. Granger E. Westberg. The various stages of grief are outlined and a constructive approach to loss is provided. A brief book to be used over and over. Fortress Press.

When There Is No Miracle by the Rev. Robert L. Wise. Comfort to believers experiencing tragedy during those times when God does not grant a miracle. Regal Books.

Changed Forever: Five Stories of God's Transforming Grace edited by the Rev. Robert DeGrandis, S.J. Testimonies of major healings. Servant Publications.

The Prayer that Heals: Praying for Healing in the Family by Dr. Francis MacNutt. A simple, helpful little book on how to pray for your loved ones. Ave Maria Press.

The Problem of Pain by C. S. Lewis. A wise, sensitive answer to the perennial question: If God is so loving and intervenes regularly in human affairs today, why is there still suffering? Macmillan.

Healing Evangelism: Strengthen Your Ministry with Effective Prayer for the Sick by the Rev. Don Dunkerley. Intentional, effective prayer for healing will strengthen the ministry of evangelism. Many practical guidelines. Chosen Books.

Resources

Here are just two of the many organizations you can contact for help in growing in your ministry of healing:

Institute for Christian Renewal. Led by the Rev. Canon Mark A. Pearson, the Institute exists to assist individuals and local churches in experiencing the riches Christ offers and in serving effectively in His name. The Institute has a variety of resources for training and equipping people in the ministry of Christian healing, and sponsors Canon Pearson as he travels to churches around the world to conduct healing missions and training programs.

You can contact the Institute at:

Institute for Christian Renewal
148 Plaistow Rd.
Plaistow, NH 03865
(603) 382-0273

The International Order of St. Luke the Physician. An international, interdenominational fellowship of clergy, medical people and laity dedicated to the ministry of Christian healing. In existence for the better part of the twentieth century, O.S.L. is considered one of the oldest and best ministries in this field.

You can contact O.S.L. at:

P.O. Box 13701
San Antonio, TX 78213
(512) 492-5222

Subject Index

Abel, 17
Abimelech, 312
Abraham, 194, 312
Adam, 16–18, 84, 131, 133, 166
Aeneas, 316
Albrecht, Mark, 125
Alcoholics Anonymous (AA),
    116–17
All Souls Church (England), 227
American Journal of Psychiatry, 157
Ananias, 316
*And Their Eyes Were Opened:
    Encountering Jesus in the Sacra-
    ments* (Scanlan and Shields), 192
Anglican Digest, The, 141
Apostolic Preaching of the Cross
    (Morris), 77
Assembly of God, 25
Augustine, Saint, 48, 196–97
Aulen, Gustav, 77

baptism, 145, 188, 189, 202; heal-
    ing power of, 193–95; Holy
    Spirit and, 193–94, 213–14,
    225; of Jesus, 143, 225
Baptist Church, 214, 236
Barnabas, 316
Barnett, Tommy, 25
Barrows, Cliff, 46

Barry, Constance P., 325
Barth, Karl, 137
Bartimaeus, 315
Baughen, Michael, 71, 227
Bennett, Dennis, 220–21
Bloom, Allan, 140
Book of Common Prayer, The, 11, 35,
    237, 321, 322, 332
Borge, Victor, 224
Buckingham, Jamie, 80
Byrd, Randolph C., 49–50, 324–27

Cain, 17
Calvin, John, 202
Catholic Church, 192, 200, 214,
    234, 304; false memory syn-
    drome and, 128; healing
    through, 19–21, 24; sacraments
    and, 193, 202, 331; saints, cult
    of the, 35–36; Vatican II, 11,
    198
Christian Medical and Dental Soci-
    ety (CMDS), 156–57
"Christian Psychiatry: The Impact
    of Evangelical Belief on Clinical
    Practice" (Galanter, Larson, and
    Rubenstone), 157
Christian Science, 178
Christus Victor (Aulen), 77

Scripture Index